Your Body's Many Cries for Water

Many illnesses which today plague millions of people worldwide spring from a simple unrecognised cause - we don't drink enough water ! When our bodies eventually cry out painfully in protest, we call these desperate thirst signals asthma, diabetes, arthritis, angina, obesity, Alzheimer's, high cholesterol and hypertension among other maladies.

This is the breakthrough medical discovery that Iranian-born Dr Batmanghelidj outlines in this extraordinary book - and if we drank more water daily, he maintains, many of the degenerative diseases could be prevented or even cured.

Dr Batmanghelidj first discovered the curative powers of water in an overcrowded Tehran prison where he was held during the 1979 revolution. One day in desperation he prescribed the only medication available for one of 3,000 terrified inmates who was literally dying of acute stomach pain - a single glass of water. The man recovered within minutes. In that moment, he asserts, 'a new era in the advancement of medical science was born.'

After his release Dr B escaped to the United States to begin further research into water as a medication. Largely ignored by the American Medical Association after presenting his findings to them nearly 20 years ago, his response was to write this book to support many meticulous, peer-reviewed scientific articles.

Your Body's Many Cries for Water has already sold over a quarter of a million copies in the United States alone. It has also been published in Iran, India, Slovenia, France and Germany. Many testimonial letters from readers and medical specialists alike included in this new British edition amply confirm the effectiveness of his method.

Dr Batmanghelidj passionately believes that if his findings were widely adopted, billions of dollars could be lopped from annual healthcare budgets in all advanced countries - greatly reducing our dependence on manufactured drugs from the giant pharmaceutical companies. But ultimately, he says, the book should be read as a love story, like a novel which describes 'the beautiful and compelling love relationship between water and the human body.'

YOUR BODY'S MANY CRIES FOR WATER

A revolutionary natural way
to prevent illness and
restore good health

Dr F Batmanghelidj

TAGMAN

www.tagman-press.com
London, Sydney, Los Angeles

YOUR BODY'S MANY CRIES FOR WATER

First simultaneous hardcover/revised paperback publication in the United
Kingdom in 2000 by The Tagman Press, an imprint of Tagman Worldwide Ltd,
Lovemore House, P O Box 754, Norwich NR1 4GY
E mail editorial@tagman-press.com

Also at :

1888 Century Park East, Suite 1900, Los Angeles, CA 90067-1702, USA.
31, Denham Street, Bondi, NSW 2026, Australia.

Initially published in USA by Global Health Solutions Inc, 1992.
Second edition 1995, reprinted 1995, 1996, 1997, 1998, 1999.
Hardcover edition 1997, reprinted 1997, 1998.

First paperback publication in the UK by The Therapist Ltd., 1994.
Second edition 1997.

Revised UK hardcover/paperback edition by The Tagman Press April 2000.
First reprint August 2000, 2nd reprint June 2001, 3rd reprint August 2001.

ISBN 0-9530921-5-1 (hardcover) 0-9530921-6-X (paperback).
A CIP catalogue record for this book is available from The British Library.

Produced for The Tagman Press by Scribble Ink
Printed in the UK by MFP Design & Print, Longford Trading Estate,
Stretford, Manchester M32 0JT.
Illustrations by Alan Baker.

TAGMAN

www.tagman-press.com

To our Creator,
with awe, humility,
dedication and love

Publisher's foreword

This first hardcover and simultaneous paperback edition of *Your Body's Many Cries for Water* is published by The Tagman Press in the United Kingdom and British Commonwealth, following earlier UK publication of paperback editions in 1994 and 1997 by The Therapist Ltd. The book was originally published in the USA in 1992 by Global Solutions Inc. Since then, it has been repeatedly reprinted in the United States, often several times each year. Translated editions have also been published in a number of European countries, including Germany and France.

All told, more than a quarter of a million copies of this remarkable and increasingly influential book have now been printed.

Since first publication, the author's revolutionary health message has remained essentially unchanged. However, for this new and revised UK edition, he has added an up-to-date postscript. It describes fully for the first time his persistent, but so far unsuccessful, efforts to persuade medical authorities in the United States and elsewhere to investigate and endorse his proven discovery of the simple curative and preventive powers of increased daily water consumption in the context of general good health and many degenerative illnesses.

From all countries where the book has been read or published to date, including the United Kingdom, many readers have written to the author describing the various health improvements they have experienced after reading his work and sharing its information with their medical advisers.

These positive responses continually provide fresh corroboration of Dr Batmanghelidj's findings. The Tagman Press strongly supports the author's efforts to make these health benefits more widely known in the UK and beyond, with a view to redirecting some of the vast medical resources currently, in the author's opinion, being wasted on unnecessary drug treatments. We will swiftly forward any letters from readers to Dr Batmanghelidj, to add to the positive store of practical personal experiences that are so valuable in expanding knowledge and promoting his unique health care message.

Anthony Grey, Summer 2001.

CONTENTS

Acknowledgements

I would like to thank my wife Xiaopo for her loving support and help. I would like to express my sincere appreciation to Colonel Robert T Sanders for his tireless efforts to make sure that my views on chronic dehydration are heard by the people he thinks might wish to help in 'spreading the message'. I would also like to thank all of those who have been exuberant supporters and have encouraged me to continue and not get tired. Finally, I would like to thank Mrs Dorothy Heindel for her editorship of all my manuscripts and books.

Introduction

After my training at St Mary's Hospital Medical School of London University and having the honour of being selected as one of the resident doctors in my own medical school, I returned to Iran, where I was born, to set up medical centres and clinics for those in need.

This endeavour became very successful – until the political volcano erupted as the angry masses engaged in the violent overthrow of the Shah and the Iranian government.

And there was a tragic side to this historic event. Almost all the professional and creative people who had stayed in the country were rounded up and taken to prison to be investigated, tried and 'dealt with' as quickly as possible. Some were shot on the first day or two. Their revolutionary trials consisted simply of establishment of identity and pronouncement of guilt, followed by sentence. The trial would last no more than ten minutes. Others were given a little more time before being 'processed'.

I was lucky to be among the latter group. I suppose my skills as a doctor were useful to the prison authorities, explaining the delay in my being processed.

Evin Prison in Tehran, where I was held for two years and seven months, was built for 600 persons. At one point, it was 'sardine-packed' with 8,000 to 9,000 people. At the height of revolutionary fervour, when segregating different political factions, the authorities used cells built for six to eight to isolate up to 90 people. One third would lie down, one third would squat and one third had to stand. Every few hours, the prisoners would rotate position.

The nightmare of life and death in that hell-hole haunted everyone and tested the mettle of both strong and weak. This was when the human body revealed to me some of its greatest secrets – secrets never understood by the medical profession.

For most of the prisoners, who ranged in age from 14 to 80, the pressures of the exceptionally harsh life caused much stress and ill health. Destiny must have chosen me to be there to help some of these desperate people. One night, about two months into my imprisonment – I had begun with six weeks in solitary confinement – that destiny revealed itself.

It was past 11 pm. I awakened to awareness of an inmate who was suffering excruciating stomach pain. He could not walk by himself. Two others were helping him stay upright. He was suffering from peptic ulcer disease and wanted medication. His face dropped when I told him I had not been allowed to bring medical supplies with me to the prison.

Then the breakthrough occurred!

I gave him two glasses of water.

His pain disappeared in minutes and he could begin to stand up by himself. He beamed from ear to ear. You cannot imagine the joy of relief he experienced, even in such harsh surroundings.

'What happens if the pain comes back?' he asked.

'Drink two glasses of water every three hours,' I replied.

He became pain-free and remained disease-free for the rest of his time in prison. His 'water cure' in that harsh environment amazed me as a doctor. I knew I had witnessed a healing power of water that I had not been taught in medical school. I felt sure that no similar observation had ever been made in medical research.

If water could cure a painful disease condition in such a stressful environment, surely it needed further research? I realised that my destiny as a healer had brought me to this 'human stress laboratory' to teach me a new approach to medicine and to reveal many other hidden secrets about the human body. I opened my eyes. Instinctively, I realised why I had ended up in prison!

I stopped thinking about myself and started to think about doing medical research. I began to identify the many health problems caused by the stress of prison. By far and away the largest number involved ulcer pains. I treated those who came to me with what proved to be the best 'natural elixir' – water. I found water could treat and cure more diseases than any other single medication I knew about.

It could even cure someone who was literally dying of pain! It was again past 11 pm. I was on my way to a sick inmate when I heard a piercing groan from a cell at the end of the corridor. I followed the sound and found a young man curled up on the floor of his cell. He seemed to be totally detached, giving out deep, piercing groans.

'What is wrong?' I asked.

He did not react. I had to shake him before he managed to reply, 'My ulcer is killing me.'

'What have you done for the pain?' I asked.

He haltingly explained, 'Since one o'clock . . . when it started . . . I have taken three Tagamets . . . one full bottle of antacid . . . but the pain has got worse since then.' (At that time, prisoners were able to get medication from the prison hospital.)

By now, I had a much clearer understanding of peptic ulcer pain. What I did not realise until then was the severity it could reach, when not even strong medication could stop it. After examining his abdomen for possible complications, I gave him two glasses of tap water – just over one pint (0.5 litre). I left him to visit another sick inmate. Ten minutes later I returned. Groans of pain no longer filled the corridor.

'How do you feel?' I asked.

'Much better,' he replied, 'but I still have some pain.'

I gave him a third glass of water. And his pain stopped completely within four minutes.

This man had been semi-conscious, on the verge of death. He had taken a huge amount of ulcer medication – with no result. And now, after drinking only three glasses of tap water, he became pain-free, sitting up and socialising with friends.

What a humbling discovery. And I thought I had received the best medical education in the world, in London!

During nearly three years of my captivity, I cured over 3,000 ulcer cases with only water in Tehran's Evin Prison – 'my God-given stress laboratory'. All thanks to water. Plain, simple, cost-free medicine for everyone. Water that we all take for granted! Water that the medical profession has dismissed as unworthy of research!

Since my eyes were opened to water as a natural medication, I have developed and applied this technique to the point where it has alleviated and healed hundreds of traditionally incurable sicknesses and chronic pains. I have seen water completely reverse conditions such as: asthma; angina; hypertension; migraine headaches; arthritis pain; back pain; colitis pain and chronic constipation; heartburn and hiatal hernia; depression; chronic fatigue syndrome; high cholesterol; morning sickness; overweight problems – even heart problems thought to need bypass surgery. All these disease conditions have responded simply and permanently to water. Ordinary 'natural' water. Any water you feel comfortable drinking is fine. Clean tap water is as good as any.

This book reveals how water can cure so many health problems, by explaining what happens when there is not enough water in the body, and contains the information you need to apply this simple but effective discovery to your own well-being.

An important note

Information and recommendations on water intake presented in this book are based on training, personal experience, very extensive research, and other publications of the author on the topic of water metabolism in the body. The author of this book does not dispense medical advice or prescribe the use or the discontinuance of any medication as a form of treatment without the advice of an attending physician, either directly or indirectly. The sole intention of the author, based on recent knowledge of micro-anatomy and molecular physiology, is to offer information on the importance of water to well-being, and to help inform the public of the damaging effects of chronic dehydration to the body – from childhood to old age.

This book is not intended to replace sound medical advice from a physician. On the contrary, sharing of the information contained in this book with the attending physician is highly desirable. Application of the information and recommendations described herein are undertaken at the individual's own risk. The adoption of the information should be in strict compliance with the instructions given here. Very sick persons with past history of major diseases and under professional supervision, particularly those with severe renal disease, should not make use of the information contained in this book without the supervision of their attending physician.

All recommendations and procedures contained herein are made without any guarantee on the part of the author or publisher, their agents or employees. Of necessity, the author and publisher disclaim all liability in connection with the use of information presented herein, which should always be used on the basis of another natural gift – sound common sense.

CHAPTER 1

Why 'medicine' does not cure disease

*Medical professionals of today do not understand
the vital roles of water in the human body:
medications are palliatives. They are not
designed to cure the degenerative
diseases of the human body.*

This book is about the role of water in the body and how a brief understanding of this topic can transform the health needs of our society – and how preventive medicine can become the main approach to health care in any society. The hero is *water*. The view of this book is that water is the primary substance and the leading agent in the routine events that take place in the human body. With the primary role of water in mind, we look at some disease conditions. The missing role of water in physiological situations that eventually become disease conditions is discussed.

In the 'diseases' that are discussed, a possible initial role of water metabolism disturbance needs to be excluded before we assume these conditions to have been caused through other processes. *This is the true meaning of a preventive approach to health care.* We should first exclude the simpler causes for disease emergence in the body and then think of the more complicated. *The simple truth is that dehydration can cause disease.* Everyone knows that water is 'good' for the body, but few seem to understand fully how essential it is to one's well-being or *what happens to the body if it does not receive its daily requirement of water.* When you have read this book, you will have a clearer understanding of this issue.

The solution for prevention and treatment of dehydration-produced diseases is water intake on a regular basis. This is what is described in this book. I discuss why, in the majority of cases, the disease conditions should be viewed as dehydration-produced disorders. If, by the simple intake of an added amount of water every day, you can get better, you do not need to worry. You should seek professional help if the adjustment to dietary needs of your body does not help and a medical problem continues to trouble you. What is being offered here is the necessary knowledge for disease prevention and cure of dehydration diseases.

At the end of the book you can find information on the necessary adjustments to daily water intake, and the complementary diet to prevent 'dehydration diseases', or *even cure them,* if a totally irreversible situation has not developed.

The basics

When the human body developed from species that were given life in water, the same dependence on the life-giving properties of water was inherited. The role of water in the body of living species – mankind included – has not changed since the first creation of life from salt water and its subsequent adaptation to fresh water.

When life on land became an objective, a gradually refined body water-preservation system had to be created for further species development. This process of temporary adaptation to transient dehydration became inherited as a well established mechanism in the human body and is now the infrastructure of all operative systems within the bodies of modern humans.

For the earlier water-dwelling species, adventure beyond their known boundaries constituted great stress in case they dried up. This 'stress' established a dominant physiology for crisis management of water. In the now 'stressed' humans, exactly the same translation and the physiology of crisis management of water becomes established. The process primarily involves a strict rationing of the water 'reserves' of the body. It is assumed that water supply for the immediate needs of the body is limited. Management of the available reserves of water in the body becomes the responsibility of a complex system.

This complex multi-level water rationing and distribution process remains in operation until the body receives unmistakable signals that it has gained access to adequate water supply. Since *every function of the body is monitored and pegged to the flow of water,* 'water management' is the only way of making sure that adequate amounts of water and its transported nutrients first reach the more vital organs that will have to confront and deal with any new 'stress'. This mechanism became more and more established for survival against natural enemies and predators. It is the ultimate operative system for survival in *fight or flight* situations. It is still the operative mechanism in the competitive environment of modern life in our society.

One of the unavoidable processes in the body water rationing phase is the cruelty with which some functions are monitored so that one structure does not receive more than its predetermined share of water. This is true for all organs of the body. Within these systems of water rationing, the brain function takes absolute priority over all the other systems. The brain is about 2 per cent of the total body weight, but it receives 18 to 20 per cent of blood circulation. When the 'ration masters' in charge of body water reserve regulation and distribution become more and more active, they also give their own alarm signals to show that the area in question is short of water, very much like the radiator of a car giving out steam when the cooling system is not adequate to drive up hill.

In advanced societies, thinking that tea, coffee, alcohol, and manufactured beverages are desirable substitutes for the natural water needs of the daily 'stressed' body is an elementary – but catastrophic – mistake. It is true that these beverages contain water, but they also contain dehydrating agents. They get rid of the water they are dissolved in, plus some more water from the reserves of the body! Modern life-styles make people dependent on all sorts of beverages that are commercially manufactured. Children are not educated to drink water; they become dependent on sodas and juices. This is a self-imposed restriction on the water needs of the body. It is not generally possible to drink manufactured beverages to completely replace the water the body needs. At the same time, a cultivated preference for the taste of these sodas automatically reduces the urge to drink water when sodas are not available, thus leading to dehydration.

Practitioners of medicine are unaware of the many chemical roles of water in the body. Because dehydration eventually causes loss of some functions, the various sophisticated signals given by operators of the body's water rationing programme during severe and lasting dehydration have been translated as indicators of unknown disease conditions of the body. *This is the most basic mistake that has deflected clinical medicine. It has stopped medical practitioners being able to advise preventive measures or offer simple physiologic cures for some of the major human diseases.*

With the appearance of these signals, the body should be provided with water for the rationing systems to distribute. However, medical practitioners have been taught to *silence* these signals with chemical products. Of course, they don't understand the significance of this gross error. The various signals produced by these water distributors are indicators of *regional thirst* and drought of the body. At the onset, they can be relieved by an increased intake of water, yet they are improperly dealt with by the use of commercial chemical products until pathology is established and diseases are born. This error continues with the use of more and more chemicals to treat other developing symptoms, the complications of dehydration become unavoidable, and then the patient dies. The irony of this is that the practitioners say the patient died of a disease!

The error in silencing the different signals of water shortages of the body with chemical products is immediately detrimental to the cells of the body. The established signal-producing chronic dehydration also has a permanently damaging impact on subsequent descendants of the person.

I take pleasure in bringing to your attention this breakthrough in medical knowledge that can benefit every person who may fall ill, and especially the elderly. In short, my paradigm change in basic human applied science will establish a physiology-based approach to future human research and simplify the practice of medicine all over the world. The immediate outcome of this paradigm shift will be to the health advantage of the public. It will expose the newly understood signs of dehydration in the human body. It will also decrease the consequent costs of illness.

The paradigm that needs to be changed

What is a paradigm and how does it change? A *paradigm* (pronounced paradime) is the most basic understanding on which new knowledge is generated. As an example, an earlier understanding was that the Earth is flat. The new understanding is that the Earth is round. The roundness of the Earth is the basic paradigm to the design of all maps, globes, recognition of stars in the sky, and calculations for space travel. Thus, the earlier paradigm for holding the Earth to be flat was inaccurate. It is the correct understanding of the Earth as a sphere that has made advancement in many fields of science possible. This change in paradigm is basic to our progress in many fields of science. The shift in that paradigm and the transformation it brought about did not occur easily. Adoption of a fundamentally significant new paradigm in the science of medicine is more difficult even if the outcome is highly desirable and desperately needed by society.

The source of error in medicine

The human body is composed of 25 per cent solid matter (the solute) and 75 per cent water (the solvent). Brain tissue is said to consist of 85 per cent water. When the phase of inquiry into the body's workings began, scientific parameters and broad knowledge of chemistry were well established, so it was automatically assumed that the same understandings that were developed within the discipline of chemistry applied to the body's solute composition.

It was therefore assumed that the solute composition is the reactive regulator of all functions of the body. At the onset of physiological research, the body's water content was assumed to act only as a solvent, space filler, and means of transport. These same views were generated from experiments in chemistry. No other functional properties were attributed to the solvent material. The basic understanding in today's 'scientific' medicine, inherited from an educational programme established at the dawn of systematic learning, also regards solutes as regulators and water as only a solvent and a means of material transport in the body. The human body is, even now, regarded as a large 'test tube' full of solids of different nature and the water in the body as a chemically insignificant 'packing material'.

In science, it has been assumed that solutes (substances dissolved or carried in the blood and serum in the body) regulate all the body's activities. This includes regulation of its water (the solvent) intake, which is assumed to be well-regulated. It is presumed, because water is freely available and one does not have to pay for it, that the body has no business in falling short of something that is so available!

Under this erroneous assumption, human applied research has been directed toward identification of one 'particular' substance that can be held responsible for causing a disease. Therefore, suspected possible fluctuations and variation of elemental changes have been tested without a clear-cut solution to a single disease problem. Accordingly, all treatments are palliative and none seems to be curative (except the use of antibiotics for bacterial infections).

Hypertension is not generally *cured;* it is *treated* during a person's lifetime. Asthma is not *cured;* inhalers are the constant companion of the afflicted. Peptic ulcers are not *cured;* antacids have to be nearby all the time. Allergy is not *cured;* the victim is always dependent on medication. Arthritis is not *cured,* it eventually cripples, and so on.

Based on this preliminary assumption of the role of water, it has become a practice to regard the dry mouth as a sign and sensation of body water needs. These needs are assumed to be well regulated if the sensation of dry mouth is not present, possibly because the substance water is abundant and free. *This is an absurdly erroneous and confusion-generating view in medicine and entirely responsible for the lack of success in finding permanent preventive solutions to disease emergence in the body, despite costly research.*

I have already published an account of my clinical observations when I treated more than 3,000 peptic ulcer sufferers with water alone. I discovered for the first time in medicine that this 'classical disease' of the body responds to water by itself. Clinically, it became obvious that this condition resembled a thirst 'disease'. Under the same environmental and clinical settings, other 'disease' conditions seemed to respond to water by itself. Extensive research has proven my clinical observations that the body has a variety of most sophisticated thirst signals – integrated signal systems during regulation of the available water at times of dehydration.

The combination of my clinical and literature research has shown that the paradigm that has until now governed all human applied research must be changed if we wish to conquer 'disease'. It has become clear that the practice of clinical medicine is based on a *false* assumption and an *inaccurate* premise. Otherwise, how could a signal system for water metabolism disturbance be missed or so blatantly ignored for such a long time? At the moment, the dry mouth is the *only* accepted sign of dehydration of the body. As I have explained, this signal is the *last* outward sign of *extreme* dehydration. *The damage occurs at a level of persistent dehydration that does not necessarily demonstrate a dry mouth signal.* Earlier researchers should have realised that, to facilitate the act of chewing and swallowing food, saliva is produced even if the rest of the body is comparatively dehydrated.

Naturally, chronic dehydration of the body means persistent water shortage that has become established for some time. Like any other deficiency disorder, such as vitamin C deficiency in scurvy, vitamin B deficiency in beri-beri, iron deficiency in anaemia, vitamin D deficiency in rickets, or you name it, the most efficient method of treatment of the associated disorders is by supplementing the missing ingredient. Accordingly, if we recognise the health complications of chronic dehydration, their prevention, and even early cure, becomes simple.

Although my scientific views in medicine were peer reviewed before I presented my paradigm change information as a guest lecturer at an international cancer conference in 1987, Dr Barry Kendler's letter overleaf (printed by his permission) further confirms the validity of my scientific views on chronic dehydration as a disease producer. As you can see, he has studied some of the important references which I have quoted to explain that chronic dehydration is the root cause of most major degenerative diseases of the human body – the causes of which were not clear until now. Referring to any medical text-book, you will see over a thousand pages of verbiage, but when it comes to giving the reasons for the major diseases of the human body, the statement in all cases is uniform and very brief: 'Aetiology unknown!'

Manhattan College

RIVERDALE, NEW YORK 10471

DEPARTMENT OF BIOLOGY
COLLEGE OF MOUNT ST. VINCENT CAMPUS

College of Mount St. Vincent

RIVERDALE, NEW YORK 10471
(212) 549-8000

6-20-94

F. Batmanghelidj, M.D.
2146 Kings Garden Way
Falls Church, VA 22043

Dear Dr. Batmanghelidj:

   I had the opportunity of reading some of your publications concerning the significance of adequate hydration and the role of chronic dehydration in the etiology of disease. While perusing this material, I carefully examined many of the references that you had cited, especially those in your paper published in Anticancer Research (1987:7:971) and in your subsequent paper in Volume 1 of Science in Medicine Simplified.

   Every reference that I checked was properly used to support your hypothesis that a paradigm shift from a solute-based to a solvent-based body metabolism is warranted. I conclude, based upon study of your revolutionary concept, that its implementation by health care professionals and by the general public, is certain to have an enormous positive impact both on well-being and on health care economics. Accordingly, I will do all that I can to publicize the importance of your findings.

Yours truly,

Barry S. Kendler, Ph.D.
Associate Professor of Biology
Manhattan College

Adjunct Faculty Member
Graduate Nutrition Program
New York Medical College

CHAPTER 2

The new paradigm

'A new scientific truth is not usually presented in a way to convince its opponents. Rather, they die off, and a rising generation is familiarised with the truth from the start.'
Max Planck

The new scientific truth and *level of thinking* about the human body that will empower people to become practitioners of preventive medicine for themselves is as follows: it is the solvent – the water content – that regulates all functions of the body, including the activity of all the solutes (the solids) that are dissolved in it. The disturbances in water metabolism of the body (the solvent metabolism) produce a variety of signals, indicating a 'system' disturbance in the particular functions associated with the water supply and its rationed regulation.

Let me repeat: every function of the body is monitored and pegged to the efficient flow of water. 'Water distribution' is the only way of making sure that not only an adequate amount of water, but its transported elements (hormones, chemical messengers and nutrients) first reach the more vital organs. Every organ producing a substance to be made available to the rest of the body will monitor its own rate and standards of production and release into the 'flowing water' according to constantly changing quotas set by the brain. Once the water itself reaches the 'drier' areas, it also exercises its many other vital and missing physical and chemical regulatory actions.

Knowing this, water intake and its priority distribution achieve paramount importance. The regulating neuro-transmitter systems (histamine and its subordinate agents) become increasingly active during the regulation of water requirements of the body. Their action should not be continuously blocked by the use of medication. Their purpose should be understood and satisfied by drinking more water.

I made these statements to a body of scientists that had gathered from all over the world in Monte Carlo in 1989 for a conference on the topic of inflammation, analgesics, and immune modulators.

The new paradigm permits incorporation of the *'fourth dimension of time'* into scientific research. It will facilitate an understanding of the damaging effect of an establishing dehydration that persists and continues to increase over any period. It will make it possible to forecast the physiological events that will lead to disease states in later years, including those which, at present, appear as genetic disorders. It will transform the present 'shot-in-the-dark, symptoms-treating' approach to the practice of medicine into a scientifically accurate medical art; it will make preventive forecasting possible. It will establish excellent health and reduce the health care costs of individuals and any society that fosters its spread.

Since water shortage in different areas of the body will manifest varying symptoms, signals, and complications now labelled 'diseases', people may think water could not be offered as a natural solution: 'Water cures so many diseases? No way!' Speaking thus, they shut their minds to the new possibility of preventing and possibly even curing so many different 'diseases' that are produced by dehydration. It does not occur to them that the only remedy for conditions that come about when the body begins to get dehydrated is water – and nothing else. A number of sample testimonials are published in this book to open the eyes of sceptics to the fact that the greatest health discovery of all times is that water is a natural medication for a variety of health conditions.

Water regulation at different stages of life

There are basically three stages to water regulation of the body in the different phases of life. One, the first stage of life of a foetus in the uterus of the mother (left of B in Figure 1 on page 21). Two, the next phase of growth until full height and width is achieved (approximately between the ages of 18 and 25). Three, the phase of life from fully grown to the demise of the person.

During the intra-uterine stage of cell expansion, water for cell growth of the child has to be provided by the mother. However, the transmitter system for water intake seems to be produced by the foetal tissue, but registers its effect on the mother. The first indicator for water needs of the foetus and the mother seems to be morning sickness during the early phase of pregnancy. *Morning sickness of the mother is a thirst signal of both the foetus and the mother.*

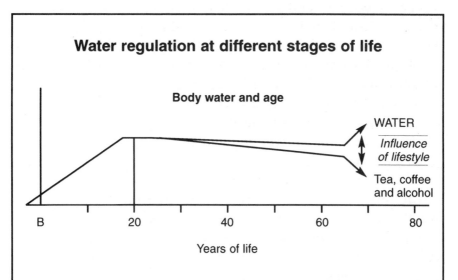

Water regulation at different stages of life

Body water and age

WATER

Influence of lifestyle

Tea, coffee and alcohol

B   20   40   60   80

Years of life

Water intake and thirst sensations

Figure 1: There are basically three stages of water regulation of the body in the different phases of life.

1   The stage of life of a foetus in the uterus of the mother (to the left of B in the diagram).

2   The phase of growth until full height and width is achieved (approximately between the ages of 18 and 25).

3   The phase of life from fully grown stage until the demise of the person. During the intra-uterine stage of cell expansion, water for cell growth of the child has to be provided by the mother.

The need for thorough understanding

It is now becoming obvious that from an early adult age, *because of a gradually failing thirst sensation,* our body becomes chronically and increasingly dehydrated. With increase in age, the water content of the cells of the body decreases, to the point that the ratio of the volume of body water that is inside the cells to that which is outside the cells changes from a figure of 1.1 and becomes almost 0.8 (see Figure 2 opposite). This is a very drastic change. Since the 'water' we drink provides for cell function and its volume requirements, the decrease in our daily water intake affects the efficiency of cell activity. It is the reason for the loss of water volume held inside the cells of the body. As a result, chronic dehydration causes symptoms that equal disease when the variety of emergency signals of dehydration are not understood. You see, these urgent cries of the body for water are treated as abnormal and dealt with by the use of medications.

The human body can become dehydrated even when water is readily available. *Humans seem to lose their thirst sensation and the critical perception of needing water. Not recognising a need for water, they gradually become increasingly and chronically dehydrated as they age* (see Figures 1 & 2). Further confusion lies in the idea that when we're thirsty tea, coffee, or alcohol-containing beverages are an adequate substitute. As you will see, this is a common error.

The dry mouth is the very last sign of dehydration. The body can suffer from dehydration even when the mouth is fairly moist. Still worse, in the elderly, the mouth can be seen to be obviously dry and yet thirst may not be acknowledged and satisfied.

Other important properties of water

Scientific research shows that water has many properties besides being a solvent and a means of transport. Failure to acknowledge the many other properties of water in the regulation of different functions in the body has produced the pitiful confusions that are the infrastructure of our so-called 'science-based' modern medicine.

Water has a firmly established and essential role in all aspects of the body's metabolic, water-dependent chemical reactions (hydrolysis), similar to the chemical powers of water that make a seed grow and

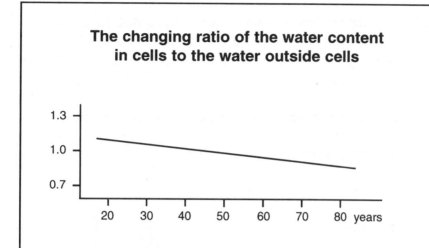

The changing ratio of the water content in cells to the water outside cells

Figure 2: *A gradual and steady loss of sensitivity of the thirst sensation and insufficient water intake will alter the ratio of the amount of water held inside all the cells to the volume of water held outside the cells of the body. The water we drink will keep the cell volume balanced and the salt we take will maintain the volume of water that is held outside the cells and in circulation.*

produce a new plant or a tree: the power of water that is used in the chemistry of life.

At the cell membrane, the osmotic flow of water through the membrane can generate *'hydroelectric' energy* (voltage gradient) that is stored in the energy pools in the form of ATP and GTP and used for elemental (cation) exchanges. ATP and GTP are chemical sources of energy in the body. The energy generated by water is used in the manufacture of ATP and GTP. These particles are used as 'cash flow' in elemental exchanges, particularly in neurotransmission.

Water also forms a particular structure, pattern and shape that seems to be employed as the *adhesive material* in bonding cell architecture. Like glue, it sticks solid structures in the cell membrane together, developing the stickiness of 'ice' at higher body temperature.

Products manufactured in the brain cells are transported on *'waterways'* to their destination in the nerve endings for use in the transmission of messages. There seem to exist small waterways or microstreams along the length of nerves that 'float' the packaged materials along 'guidelines', called microtubules (see Figure 3).

Proteins and the enzymes of the body function more efficiently in solutions of lower viscosity; this is true of all the receptors

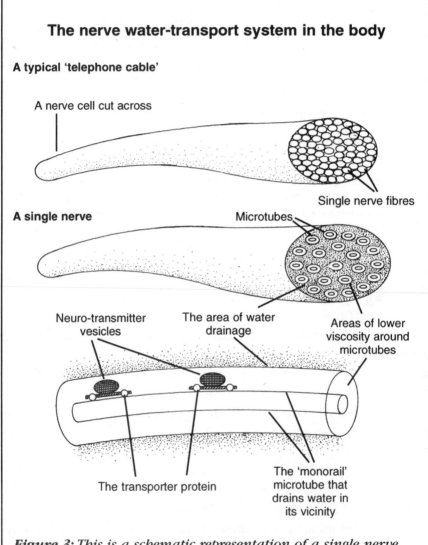

The nerve water-transport system in the body

A typical 'telephone cable'

A nerve cell cut across

Single nerve fibres

A single nerve

Microtubes

Neuro-transmitter vesicles

The area of water drainage

Areas of lower viscosity around microtubes

The transporter protein

The 'monorail' microtube that drains water in its vicinity

Figure 3: This is a schematic representation of a single nerve fibre and the waterway system of transport along the lines of microtubes that act as drainage pipes and create areas of lower viscosity v drawing water from the surrounding areas.

(receiver points) in cell membranes. In solutions of higher viscosity (in a dehydrated state), proteins and enzymes become less efficient (this possibly includes recognition of thirst of the body). It follows that water regulates all functions of the body, including the activity of all solutes it carries around.

The new scientific truth (paradigm shift): *'Water, the solvent of the body, regulates all functions, including the activity of the solutes it dissolves and circulates'* should become the basis of all future approaches to medical research.

When the body is dehydrated, apart from establishment of a 'locked-in' drive for water intake, a rationing and distribution system for the available water in the body becomes operative according to a pre-determined priority programme – a form of *drought management.*

It is now scientifically clear that the *histamine* directed and operated neurotransmitter system becomes active and initiates the subordinate systems that promote water intake. These subordinate systems also redistribute the amount of water in circulation or that can be drawn away from other areas. Subordinate systems employ *vasopressin* (vayso-press-in), *renin-angiotensin* (RA), *prostaglandins* (prosta-glan-dins, PG) and *kinins* (ky-nins) as the intermediary agents. Since the body does not have a reserve of water to draw on, it operates a priority distribution system for the amount of water that is already available or has been supplied by its intake.

In amphibians, it has been shown that histamine reserves and their rate of generation are at minimal levels. In the same species, histamine generation becomes established and is pronounced when the animal is dehydrated. Proportionate increase in the production rate and storage of neurotransmitter histamine for rationing regulation of the available water in dehydrated animals' drought management becomes established. Histamine and its subordinate water intake and distribution regulators, *prostaglandins, kinins,* and *PAF* (another histamine associated agent) also cause pain when they come across pain-sensing nerves in the body.

The above 'view shift' in medicine establishes two major points that have been disregarded until now. One, the body can become dehydrated as we get older, and it *disregards dry mouth as the only indicator of body thirst.* Two, when the neurotransmitter histamine generation and its subordinate water regulators become excessively active, to the point of causing allergies, asthma and chronic pains in different parts of the body, these pains should be translated as a thirst signal – that is, one variety of the crisis signals of water shortage in the body. This 'paradigm shift' now makes it possible to recognise many different associated signals of general or local body dehydration.

The adoption of the 'view shift' (new paradigm) dictates that chronic pains of the body, that cannot be easily explained as injury or infection, should *first and foremost* be interpreted as signals of chronic water shortage in the area where pain is registered – a local thirst. These pain signals should be first considered and excluded as primary indicators for dehydration of the body before any other complicated procedures are forced on the patient. *Non-infectious 'recurring' or chronic pains should be viewed as indicators of body thirst.*

Not recognising the body's thirst signals will undoubtedly produce complicated problems in the present way of treating these conditions. It is all too easy to assume these signals are complications of a serious disease process and begin to treat signal-producing dehydration with complicated procedures. Although water by itself will alleviate the condition, medications or invasive diagnostic procedures may be forced on the person. *It is the responsibility of both patients and their doctors to be aware of the damage that chronic dehydration can cause in the human body.*

These chronic pains include *dyspeptic pain, rheumatoid arthritis pain, anginal pain* (heart pain on walking, or even at rest), *low back pain, intermittent claudication pain* (leg pain on walking), *migraine* and *hangover headaches, colitis pain and its associated constipation* (see figure 4 opposite).

The 'view shift' dictates that all these pains should be treated with a regular adjustment to daily water intake. No less than two and a half quarts (two and one half litres) in 24 hours should be taken for a few days prior to the routine and regular use of analgesics or other pain-relieving medications such as anti-histamine or antacids – well before permanent local or general damage can be established and

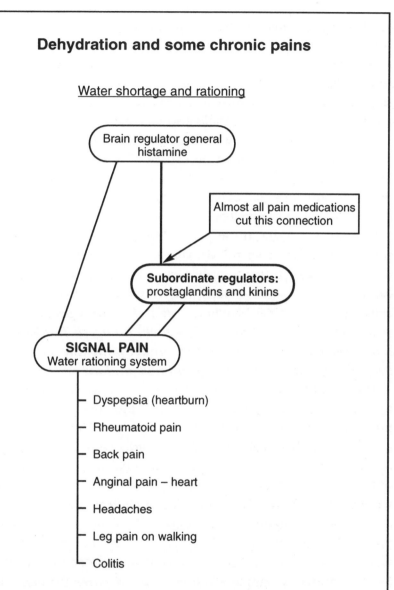

Dehydration and some chronic pains

Water shortage and rationing

Brain regulator general histamine

Almost all pain medications cut this connection

Subordinate regulators: prostaglandins and kinins

SIGNAL PAIN Water rationing system

– Dyspepsia (heartburn)

– Rheumatoid pain

– Back pain

– Anginal pain – heart

– Headaches

– Leg pain on walking

– Colitis

Figure 4: There are two components to the sensation of pain. One is local and the other is central-nervous-system-registered. At an early phase, the locally registered pain can be alleviated with painkillers. After a certain threshold is reached, the brain becomes the direct centre for monitoring its perpetuation until hydration of the body takes place.

reach an irreversible disease status. *If the problem has persisted for many years, those who wish to test the pain relieving property of water should make sure their kidneys can make sufficient urine so that they do not retain too much water in the body.* Urine output should be measured against water intake. With an increase in water intake, the urine output should also increase.

This new understanding of the *physiology of pain production in dehydration* will shed light on causes of disease in future medical research. It exposes the long-term use of pain medications for 'killing' a cardinal signal of chronic and local dehydration of the body as detrimental to the well-being of the body.

In their own right, these pain-killers (analgesics) can cause fatal side-effects, apart from the damage that is caused by the on-going dehydration that is temporarily silenced without removing the root cause of these pains – that is, dehydration. Very often, analgesics cause gastrointestinal bleeding. *A few thousand people die every year from this complication of frequent analgesic intake. By 1996, it had become clear that over-the-counter pain-killers can, in some people, cause liver and kidney damage and act as people killers.*

The scientific background for the above views is already available to scientists in pain research. This brief is intended to brush aside the professional resistance of the AMA (American Medical Association) and the NIH (National Institute of Health) which are aware of my findings but have refused to propagate them to the ultimate benefit of the public. This 'view shift' on the role of water in the body can work wonders in the future practice of clinical medicine.

The moment medical professionals adopt this paradigm shift, the present form of 'ignorance of the human body based medical practice' will transform to a thoughtful, preventive approach to health care. More importantly, simple *physiology-based cures* for early disease emergence will become available well *before* irreversible damage can be established.

CHAPTER 3

Dyspeptic pain

*A newly recognised emergency thirst signal
of the human body.*

Dyspeptic pain is the most important signal for the human body. It
denotes dehydration. It is a thirst signal of the body. It can occur in
the very young as well as older people. Chronic and persistently
increasing dehydration is the root cause of almost all currently
encountered major diseases of the human body.

Of the dyspeptic pains, that of gastritis, duodenitis, and heartburn
should be treated with an increase in water intake alone. When there
is associated ulceration, attention to the daily diet to enhance the
rate of repair of the ulcer site becomes necessary.

According to Professor Howard Spiro of Yale University, it is
generally understood that 12 per cent of those with dyspepsia develop
ulceration in their duodenum after six years, 30 per cent after 10
years and 40 per cent after 27 years. It is the dyspeptic pain that is
of significance, although the condition develops importance once
the ulceration is viewed through the endoscopic examination. It
seems that medical practice is becoming more and more a visually
oriented discipline rather than the perceptive and thought-based art
that it was at one time.

It is the pain associated with these differently classified conditions
that forces the person to consult a medical practitioner. It is this pain
that is now getting much attention, even though much jargon is
attached to the local conditions seen through the endoscope. The
common factor is the dyspeptic pain. The local tissue change is the
descriptive explanation for the changes brought about by the basic
common factor, namely the initiating dehydration.

How am I able to make such claims? In that Iranian prison, as I've
already indicated, I treated *with water only* over three thousand people

with dyspeptic pain who had other distinguishing characteristics to classify them according to the jargon mentioned above. *They all responded to an increase in their water intake, and clinical problems associated with the pain disappeared.* The report of my new method of treating dyspeptic pain with water was published as the editorial article in the *Journal of Clinical Gastroenterology* in June of 1983.

At a certain threshold of dehydration, when the body urgently calls for water, nothing else can be a substitute. No medication other than water is effective. One of the many patients I treated with water stands out and proves this fact. He was a young man in his middle twenties. He had suffered from peptic ulcer disease for a number of years before the crisis time when I met him in the prison. He had the usual diagnostic procedures performed on him and received the diagnostic label of duodenal ulcer. He had been given antacids and brand name cimetidine medications.

Cimetidine is a very strong form of medication that blocks the action of histamine on its 'second' type receiver points, generally known as receptors in the body, and, in this case, known as histamine 2 or H_2 receptors. It just happens that some cells in the stomach that produce the acid are sensitive to this medication. However, many other cells in the body that do *not* produce acid are also sensitive to this blocking action of the medication. That is why this medication has many other side effects (including impotence in the young), and has proven extremely dangerous in the chronically dehydrated older age group.

As I mentioned in my Introduction to this edition, the first time I set eyes on one young man was at eleven o'clock one evening in the summer of 1980. He was in such pain that he was almost becoming semiconscious. He was lying folded in the foetal position on the floor of his room. He was groaning, unaware of his environment and the worried people around him. When I talked to him, he did not respond. He was not communicating with those around him. I had to shake him to get a response. I asked him what was the matter.

He gasped, 'My ulcer is killing me.' I asked him how long he had been experiencing the pain. He said his pain started at one in the afternoon, immediately after his lunch. The pain increased in intensity as time passed. I asked him what he had done to get relief and if he had taken any medication. He replied that he had taken three tablets of cimetidine and one whole bottle of antacid during this time. He indicated that it had given him no relief – even with that amount of medication – in the 10 hours since his pain first started.

When so much medication cannot relieve the pain of peptic ulcer disease, one automatically becomes suspicious of 'acute abdomen', something that might possibly need surgical exploration. Maybe his ulcer had perforated! I had seen and assisted in operations on patients with perforated peptic ulcers. Those people were devastated, very much like the young man before me. The test is simple: such patients develop a very rigid abdominal wall, almost like a wooden board. I felt for the rigidity of the wall of the abdomen in this young man. Fortunately, he had not perforated. His abdominal wall was soft, but tender from the pain. He was lucky he had not perforated, although, if he had continued like this, the acid would have punched a hole through his now-inflamed ulcer.

The arsenal of medications in such circumstances is very limited. Three cimetidine tablets of 300 milligrams each and one full bottle of antacid could not relieve the pain. Often, such cases would end on the operating table of a knife-happy surgeon. Because of my extensive experience with the pain-relieving property of water in dyspeptic pains, I gave this man two full glasses of water – one pint. At first he was reluctant to drink the water. I told him he had taken the usual medications without any result. He should now try my 'medication' for this disease. He had no choice. He was in severe pain and did not know what to do about it. I sat in a corner and observed him for a few minutes.

I had to leave the room and, when I returned in about 15 minutes, his pain had become less severe and his groans stopped. I gave him another full glass of water – half a pint. In a few minutes, his pain disappeared completely and he started taking notice of the people around him. He sat up and began to move towards the wall of the room. With his back to the wall, he started to conduct conversations with his visitors who were now more surprised than he at the sudden transformation that three glasses of water had brought about! For 10 hours, this man had suffered from pain and taken the most potent and advanced medicines for the treatment of peptic ulcer disease without any relief. Now, three glasses of water had produced obvious and absolute relief in about 20 minutes.

If you refer back to Figure 4 and compare statements in the model on pain with the experience of the above patient, you will recognise the brain component to the intensity of signalling *thirst in the body*. After a certain threshold, local painkillers will not be effective. The antacid and H_2 blocking agent cimetidine did not produce even a reduction in the pain felt by the young man. It was *water alone* that registered the right message with the brain to abort its call for water, since there was now an unmistakable signal of its adequate presence in the body. The same mode of pain registration is operative in other regions that signal dehydration in any particular individual. People with rheumatoid joint pain should be aware of this phenomenon of pain registration at the brain when there is severe dehydration.

In the Iranian prison, I had another occasion to test whether the abdominal pain registration for dehydration was time-dependent or water-volume-dependent. This time, a man was carried by two other persons into the clinic where I was working at the time. The patient could not walk; he was lifted from under his arms by two other persons. He, too, was a peptic ulcer patient in extremely severe upper abdominal or dyspeptic pain. After examination to see that he had not perforated, I gave the patient one full glass of water every hour. He did not achieve total relief in 20 minutes, or even one hour and 20 minutes. He recovered after he had taken three glasses of water. On average, it takes less severe cases about *eight minutes* to achieve total pain relief.

It has been shown experimentally that, when we drink one glass of water, it *immediately* passes into the intestine and is absorbed. However, within 30 minutes, almost the same amount of water is secreted into the stomach through its glandular layer in the mucosa. It swells from underneath and gets into the stomach, ready to be used for food breakdown. The act of digestion of solid foods depends on the presence of copious amounts of water. The acid is poured on the food, enzymes are activated, and the food is broken down into a homogenised fluid state that can pass into the intestine for the next phase of digestion.

The mucus covers the glands' layer of the mucosa, which is the innermost layer of the structure of the stomach (see Figure 5 overleaf). Mucus consists of 98 per cent water and 2 per cent of the physical 'scaffolding' that traps water. In this 'water layer', called the 'mucous layer', a natural buffer state is established. The cells below secrete sodium bicarbonate that becomes trapped in the water layer. As the acid from the stomach tries to go through this protective layer, the bicarbonate neutralises it.

The outcome of this action is a greater production of salt (sodium from the bicarbonate and chlorine from the acid). Too much salt alters the water-holding properties of the 'scaffolding' material of mucus. Too much acid neutralisation and salt deposits in this mucous layer would make it less homogeneous and sticky, thus allowing the acid to get to the mucosal layer, causing pain.

The natural design in the resecretion of water through the mucous layer seems to be the process of *'back-washing'* the mucous layer and getting rid of the salt deposits. This is a most efficient design for rehydrating the mucous layer from the bottom when new mucus is also secreted. This refreshed, thickened and sticky mucous barrier is the natural protective shield against the acid in the stomach. Naturally, the efficiency of this shield depends on a regular intake of water, particularly before the intake of different solid foods that would stimulate the production of acid from glands in the stomach wall. Thus, water provides the only natural protection against the acid in the stomach, from base upward. Antacids are designed to attach to the acid in the stomach – an inefficient protection.

We should begin to realise that, in the same way as we have a hunger pain signal, we also have a thirst pain signal in the body. It is very unfortunate that it is called dyspepsia and treated with all sorts of medications until there is local duodenal or stomach tissue damage from metabolic complications of dehydration. The use of antacids for the relief of this pain is generally the accepted form of treatment. These substances are non-prescription slow poisons.

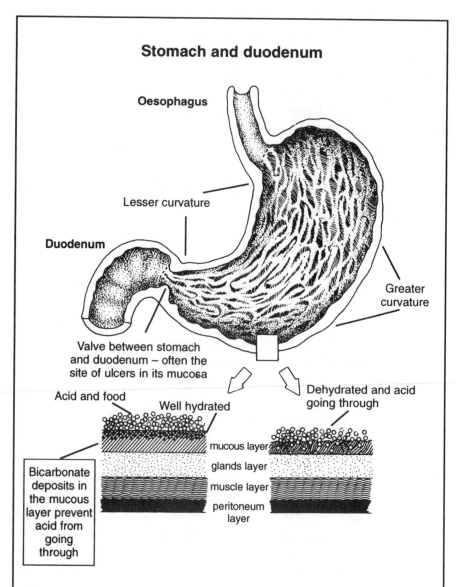

Figure 5: *A model of the stomach and its mucosal structures. A well hydrated mucous barrier retains bicarbonate and neutralises the acid as it tries to pass through the mucus. A dehydrated body also predisposes to an inefficient mucous barrier that permits acid penetration and mucosal damage. Hydration provides a much better acid barrier to the mucosa than any medication on the market.*

Significant research conducted in Sweden has shown that *the outcome is the same* in people who do not have an actual ulcer and yet have the classical dyspeptic pain, whether or not they use a placebo, an antacid, or even the agent that blocks the action of histamine. In other words, neither antacid nor the stronger medication are particularly effective. It is at this stage of body physiology, now generating signals of dehydration, that one should be prudent and refrain from the use of any form of medication.

Water is most probably the only effective substance to give relief. After all, water, and only water, is what the body *wants, needs,* and *is calling for.* If we search accurately for other signs, there would be more indicators of dehydration. Do not imagine that dyspeptic pain is the indicator of an isolated and localised phenomenon. *In any case, dyspeptic pain is a signal of dehydration - a thirst signal - of the body, even if there is an associated ulcer.* If water is taken and it relieves your pain, with adequate food intake, the ulcer should repair itself in due time.

It is now said that ulcers are the result of infections. My researched opinion is that the variety of curved bacteria, called helicobacters, blamed for causing ulcerations, are commensals - that is, bacteria that naturally dwell in the intestines. They may take unfair advantage of the immune system suppression that is the direct outcome of dehydration. You see, the normal intestinal bacteria cohabit with us and produce much of the vitamin support needed by the body. They contribute to our well-being when we are strong. In dehydration, particularly at the site of the valve between the stomach and the duodenum, many histamine producing nerves exist. This particular curved bacterium benefits from the *growth hormone effects of histamine,* at the same time that these nerves are restrictively monitoring the rate of flow of the strongly acidic content of the stomach into the intestine. In any case, not all ulcer sites show the presence of helicobacters. Also, an infinite number of people may have helicobacters in their intestines and not suffer from ulcers!

Antacids that contain aluminium are dangerous. They should not be freely used for a condition that will respond to an increase in water intake. Excessive aluminium in the circulation has been strongly implicated as a precipitating factor – with other considerations – in Alzheimer-type disease. It is imperative to understand the relationship between taking aluminium-containing antacids for a long period of time and the possible accumulative toxic side effect of brain damage in Alzheimer's disease. No amount of genetic study will undo the toxic side effect of a metal used in medications to deal with a simple signal of thirst under a wrong paradigm. Most antacids contain between 150–600 milligrams of aluminium in every spoonful of the liquid, or in each tablet.

The island of Guam has much aluminium ore in its soil (this is normally the case for some regions in the Western Pacific such as Guam island, Kii peninsula in Japan, Western New Guinea, and others). The drinking water of the island was heavily contaminated with aluminium. During the time that this contamination was not recognised and remained in the drinking water, a disease similar to Alzheimer dementia was prevalent on the island. Even the younger people on the island seemed to suffer from the disease. A number of years ago this problem was recognised and the water purified. It has been noticed that the younger people do not seem to be afflicted any more. It is now taken for granted that it was the aluminium toxicity in the drinking water that caused an Alzheimer-type of dementia on the island of Guam.

Histamine blocking agents are also not suitable for long-term use. They have many side effects. These include dizziness and confusion states in the elderly. Enlarged breasts appear in men after a few weeks of taking this medication. Low sperm count in some male patients and loss of libido have also been noted. Nursing mothers or pregnant women should not use this type of medication to treat the thirst signals of the body – the child's and the mother's. Our brain capillaries respond to dehydration by dilating if histamine stimulates them. These antihistamines will block the capillary dilating action of histamine when the brain has to tabulate more information than normal, for instance when under the pressure of stress. The brain will get less blood supply when antihistamines are used for dyspeptic pain treatment.

In my opinion, the primary cause of Alzheimer's disease is chronic dehydration of the body. I therefore believe that brain cell dehydration is the primary cause of Alzheimer's disease. Aluminium toxicity is in fact a secondary complication of dehydration in areas of the world with comparatively aluminium-free water. Caution: in the technically advanced Western societies, aluminium sulphate is, at times, used in the process of water purification for delivery into the city water supplies.

But in prolonged dehydration, the brain cells begin to shrink! Imagine a plum gradually turning into a prune! Unfortunately, in a dehydrated state, many functions of brain cells begin to get lost, such as the transport system that delivers neurotransmitters to nerve endings. One of my medical friends took this information to heart and started treating his brother, who has Alzheimer's disease, by forcing him to take more water every day. His brother has begun to recover his memory, so much so that he can now follow conversations and not frequently repeat himself. The improvement became noticeable in a matter of weeks.

Although pain is localised around the stomach, dehydration is established all over the body. Not recognising dyspeptic pain to be a thirst signal calling for water will, later in life, cause the human body many irreversible problems. Of course, a stomach tumour could cause a similar pain. However, that pain will not disappear with water. It will continue to recur. In case there are repeated pains, even when water intake has been regulated for a number of days, it would be prudent to consult a physician for assessment of the condition. If the pain is from gastritis and duodenitis, or even peptic ulcerations, regular intake of water is a must in the daily routine, as well as dietary adjustments for the treatment of the condition.

Colitis pain

Colitis pain, felt in the lower left part of the abdomen, should initially be viewed as another thirst signal for the human body. It is often associated with constipation, itself caused by persistent dehydration.

One of the main functions of the large intestine is the process of taking water out of the excrements so that too much of it is not lost in the waste matter after food digestion. When there is dehydration, the residue is naturally devoid of the normal amount of water that is necessary for its easier passage. Also, by slowing down the flow and further squeezing the content, even the final drops of water will be drawn away from the solid residue in the large gut. Thus, constipation will become a complication of dehydration in the body. With added food intake, more solid waste will be packed into the intestine and increase the burden for passage of its hardened waste content. This process will cause pain. Colitis pain should initially be considered as a thirst signal of the body. With adequate water intake, the left lower abdominal pain that is associated with constipation will disappear. Eating an apple, a pear, or an orange in the evenings helps reduce constipation the next day.

False appendicitis pain

A severe pain can sometimes appear on the right lower abdominal region. It can mimic an inflammation of the appendix and present some similarity to the pain of early appendicitis. Other distinguishing characteristics are not seen; there is no rise in body temperature; there is no guarding and tenderness in the abdominal wall and no feeling of nausea.

One or two glasses of water will relieve this lower right abdominal pain. A single glass of water can serve as a diagnostic tool for this particular condition.

Hiatus hernia

You often come across the classical dyspeptic pain that the doctor has diagnosed as hiatus hernia. Hiatus hernia means displacement of the upper part of the stomach through the gap of the diaphragm (the oesophageal hiatus) into the chest cavity. This is an unnatural location for the stomach to be in. With a part of the stomach in the chest, food digestion becomes painful.

Normally, the content of the stomach's upper part is sealed off and cannot pass upward into the oesophagus when food is being digested. The normal direction of intestinal contractions is downward, from the mouth to the rectum. Furthermore, there are two valves to prevent the regurgitation of food upward. One valve is located in the wall of the tract between the oesophagus and the stomach. This valve only relaxes when food is going into the stomach.

The other trap valve is located outside of the tract in the diaphragm, where the oesophagus passes through its hiatus to join the stomach. This 'trap valve' is synchronised to relax every time the food that is being swallowed in the oesophagus has to pass through it. At other times, it is tight and does nòt permit the content of the stomach to pass upward. This is the normal state of affairs for the two valves that prevent the passage of food from reversing direction and passing upward.

The intestinal tract, from the mouth to the rectum, is a long tube. Different parts of it have developed special physical and functional attributes to make the process of food digestion and the evacuation of its waste products a well integrated and smooth operation. There are many local hormones that make this operation possible. Local hormones are chemical messengers that signal and time the next stage of the process to 'kick in'. They cause the necessary enzymes to be secreted to further the breakdown and subsequent absorption of the active materials in food.

Early in the process of digestion, acid is secreted in the stomach to activate the enzymes and help in the breakdown of solid proteins such as meat and hard-to-digest foods. Normally, the liquefied but highly acidic content of the stomach is pumped into the first part of the intestine.

There is a valve between the stomach and the intestine, called the pyloric valve. The operation of this valve is regulated by the message system from either side of the 'tract'. It is one thing for the stomach to wish to empty its content into the intestine; it is another thing for the intestine to be ready to receive this highly corrosive and acidic gastric content.

The pancreas is a gland that secretes insulin to regulate blood sugar. It also pours essential digestive enzymes into the intestine. The pancreas has, at the same time, the physiological responsibility of rendering the intestinal environment alkaline before the acid from the stomach can reach the intestine. The most important function of the pancreas is its constant role of manufacturing and secreting a watery bicarbonate solution – the alkaline solution that will neutralise the acid that enters the intestine. To manufacture watery bicarbonate solution, the pancreas will need much water from the circulation. In dehydration, this process is not very efficient. For this reason, the pyloric valve will not receive the clear signals to open and allow stomach acid to pour into the intestine. This is the first step in the production of the dyspeptic pain, the initial thirst indicator of the human body.

When we drink water, depending on the volume of water that enters the stomach, a hormone/neurotransmitter called motilin is secreted. The more water we drink, the more motilin is produced by the intestinal tract, and can be measured in blood circulation. The effect of motilin on the intestinal tract, as its name implies, is to produce rhythmic contractions of the intestines – peristalsis – from its upper parts to its lower end. Part of this action would involve the timely opening and closing of the valves that are in the way of flow of the intestinal content.

Thus, when there is enough water in the body for all the digestive processes that depend on the availability of water, the pancreas will produce its watery bicarbonate solution to prepare the upper part of the intestinal tract to receive the acidic content of the stomach. Under such ideal circumstances, the pyloric valve is also allowed to open for the evacuation of the content of the stomach. Motilin has a major transmission role in co-ordinating this action. Motilin is a satiety hormone secreted when water extends the stomach wall.

The problem begins when there is not enough water in the body for these digestive events to take place in a co-ordinated manner. In no way will the system allow the stomach's corrosive acid content to reach the intestine if the mechanism designed to neutralise it is not effective. The damage would be irreparable. The walls of the intestines do not possess the same protective layer against acid that is available to the stomach. The first thing that happens is the reversal of the strength of contraction in the valves on either side of the stomach. The pyloric valve will constrict more and more.

The ring valve between the oesophagus and the stomach and the external 'valve' of the diaphragm will become more relaxed. Initially, some of the acid may flow into the oesophagus when the person is lying down and produce a type of pain that is often called heartburn.

In some, the laxity of the valve in the diaphragm may be such that a portion of the stomach may pass through it into the chest and achieve the title of hiatus hernia. When the valves reverse their mode of operation for the normal flow of the stomach content, in effect they are preparing for another eventual and unavoidable outcome: the evacuation of stomach content through the mouth.

If the stomach content cannot go into the intestine and it cannot indefinitely remain in the stomach, there is only one other way out – through the mouth. For this action to take place, the intestinal tract is capable of reversing the direction of its contractions. This reversal of the contractions is called anti-peristalsis.

One of the most misunderstood and upsetting conditions that is a complication of severe dehydration is *bulimia*. People who suffer from bulimia experience constant 'hunger'. After eating, they cannot retain the food and have an uncontrollable urge to vomit – thus, their antisocial lifestyle. In these people, their sensation of 'hunger' is in fact an indicator of thirst, and their urge to vomit is the protection mechanism that is explained above. If bulimics begin to rehydrate the body well and drink water before taking food, this problem should start to disappear.

In my opinion, because of the repeated corrosive effect of the regurgitating acid on the unprotected oesophageal tissue, there is a strong relationship between heartburn in early life and eventual cancer of the lower end of the oesophagus.

Dyspeptic pain, no matter what other pathological label is attached to it, should be treated by regular intake of water. Current treatment practice and the use of antacids and histamine-blocking agents is not to the benefit of a chronically dehydrated person whose body has resorted to crying for water.

A B is a woman involved in the promotion of alternative medicine, who is very strongly into chelation therapy. She has compiled other people's information and written a popular book on the subject. However, she had herself suffered for many years from excruciating pains from her hiatus hernia. Her husband tells me that A B could hardly sit through a meal; she suffered from such severe pains that she couldn't complete it. At times, they would have to leave the restaurant because the pain would not allow her even a short respite to finish her meal.

A B tells me she hardly drank any water. Only after her husband had, by chance, come across my book and read it did they finally understand A B's problem. She began drinking water. As she increased her water intake, she noticed her pain was less severe. In a matter of days it disappeared completely, never to come back. The husband and wife now enjoy going out to eat. My wife and I ate with them a few times. It appears her hiatus hernia and its pain are ancient history.

It is interesting to note that even chelation, her pet treatment procedure for so many conditions, could not help her. It should become clear that the hidden merits of chelation therapy in *most cases* is in its required high volume water intake during the actual treatment procedure. However, in the past, increased water intake was not normally a routine recommendation for the periods between treatment sessions. But, as a result of my talks and reviews of my book in their favourite *Journal of Townsend Letter for Doctors,* most practitioners of alternative medicine are now recommending increased water intake by their patients. Chelation therapy is most effective in extracting toxic metals out of the body.

In summary: dyspeptic pain is a thirst signal associated with chronic or severe dehydration in the human body. It could also exist in conjunction with other thirst pains of the body. Take a look at the letter of the radio talk show director, Samuel Liguori, on page 86. As you will see, he had both the pain of hiatus hernia and also anginal pain. With increased water intake, one pain has disappeared and the other has diminished significantly in only one week of increased water intake. At the time of the final writing of this page, his pain seemed to have cleared up completely.

CHAPTER 4

Rheumatoid arthritis pain

'The worst sin toward our fellow creatures
is not to hate them, but to be indifferent
to them: that's the essence of inhumanity.'
George Bernard Shaw

In the United States, about 50 million people suffer from some form
of arthritis, 30 million people suffer from low back pain, millions suffer
from arthritic neck pains, and 200,000 children are affected by the
juvenile form of arthritis. In Britain, an estimated 20 million people
suffer with joint symptoms, of whom four million are disabled
because of arthritis. In addition to this, in any year, a further 20 million
will have to endure back pain, with effects which range from slight
inconvenience to complete incapacity.

Once any of these conditions is established in an individual, it
becomes a sentence for suffering during the rest of the individual's
life *unless* the simplicity of problem's root-cause is fully understood.
Initially, rheumatoid arthritic joints and their pain are to be viewed
as indicators of water deficiency in the affected joint cartilage surfaces.
Arthritis pain is another of the regional thirst signals of the body. In
some arthritis pains, salt shortage may be a contributing factor.

The cartilage surfaces of bones in a joint contain much water. The
lubricating property of this 'held water' is utilised in the cartilage,
allowing the two opposing surfaces to glide freely over one another
during joint movement.

Whereas bone cells are immersed in calcium deposits, cartilage
cells are immersed in a matrix containing much water. As the cartilage
surfaces glide over one another, some exposed cells die and peel
away. New cells take their place from the growing ends that are
attached to the bone surfaces on the two sides. In a well hydrated
cartilage, the rate of friction damage is minimal. In a dehydrated
cartilage, the rate of abrasive damage is increased. The ratio between

Finger joint

Water held in the cartilage of a joint is the lubricant that protects the contact surfaces of the joint.

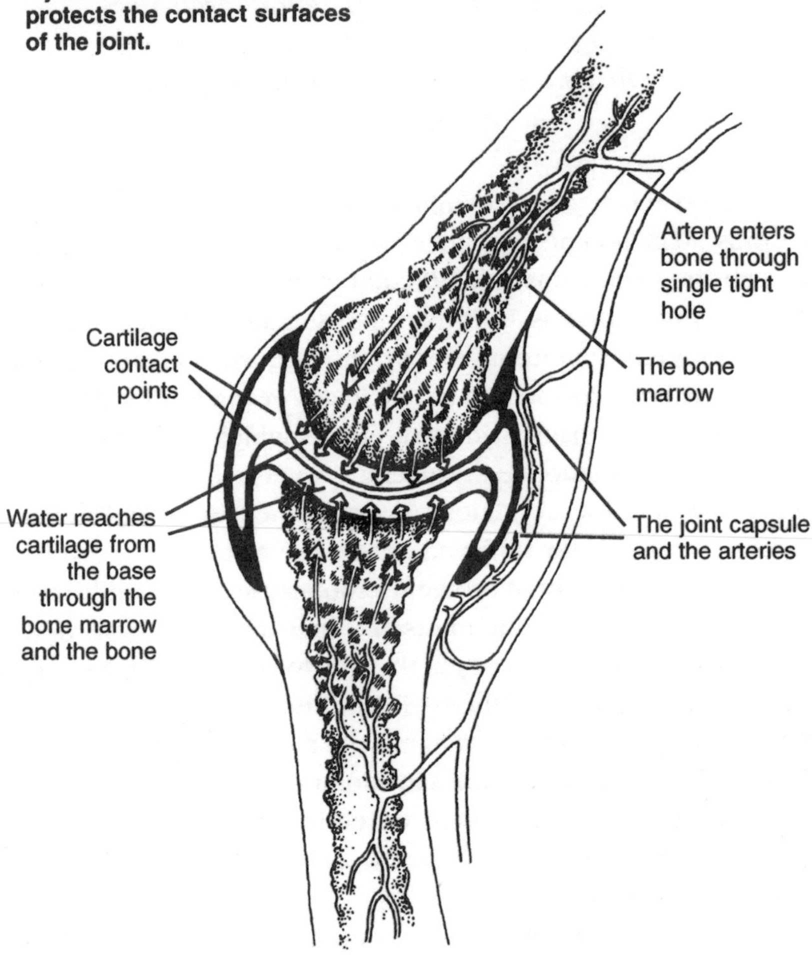

Cartilage contact points

Water reaches cartilage from the base through the bone marrow and the bone

Artery enters bone through single tight hole

The bone marrow

The joint capsule and the arteries

Figure 6: A schematic model of a normal hinge joint (found in the fingers) - its arterial supply to the bone marrow and to its capsule and the direction of serum supply to its cartilage points through the bone marrow.

the rate of regeneration of cartilage cells to their 'abrasive peel' is the index of joint efficiency.

Actively growing blood cells in the bone marrow take priority over the cartilage for the available water that goes through the bone structure. In the process of dilating the blood vessels to bring more circulation to the area, it is possible that the branch that goes through a tight hole in the bone cannot expand adequately enough to cope; the cells that depend on these vessels for an increased water and nutrient supply are under a physically imposed rationing control. Under such circumstances, and unless there is blood dilution to carry more water, the serum requirements of the cartilage will have to be satisfied from the blood vessels that feed the capsule of the joint. The nerve regulated shunting mechanisms (to all the joints) also produce signals of pain.

Initially, this pain indicates that the joint is not fully prepared to endure pressure until it is fully hydrated. This type of pain has to be treated with a regular increase in water intake to produce some dilution of blood that is circulating to the area, until the cartilage is fully hydrated and repaired from its base attachment to the bone – the normal bone route of serum diffusion to the cartilage. A look at Figures 6 (left) and 7 (overleaf) will help make these points clear.

It is my assumption that the swelling and pain in the capsule of the joint is an indication there is dilation and oedema from the vessels that furnish circulation to the capsule of the joint. Joint surfaces have nerve endings that regulate all functions. When they place a demand for more blood circulation to the area to pick up water from the serum, the compensatory vascular expansion in the capsule is supposed to make up for the inefficiency of circulation from the bone route of supply.

Because dehydration in the joint surfaces will eventually cause severe damage – to the point of making the bone surfaces bare and exposed until osteoarthritis becomes established – the tissue damage will trigger a mechanism for remodelling of the joint. There are hormone-secreting cells in the capsule of the joint. When there is damage (also from dehydration), injured tissue has to be repaired. These local remodelling hormones take over and restructure the

A comparison between a well hydrated and a dehydrated joint

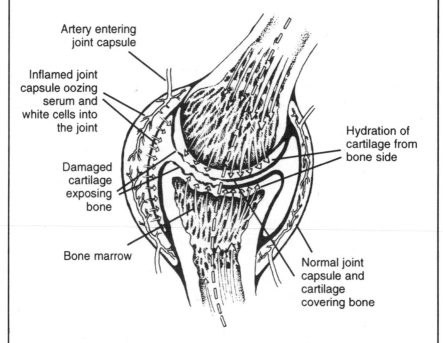

A dehydrated joint

A well hydrated joint

Artery entering joint capsule

Inflamed joint capsule oozing serum and white cells into the joint

Hydration of cartilage from bone side

Damaged cartilage exposing bone

Bone marrow

Normal joint capsule and cartilage covering bone

Joint movement causes a vacuum to be created in the joint space. Water will be pulled through the bone and the cartilage into the joint cavity – if it is freely available.

Figure 7: A schematic model intended to show and compare, side-by-side, a well hydrated joint and a dehydrated joint. The articular cartilage in a well hydrated joint gets its nutrition from the blood supply to its base attachment to the bone. A dehydrated joint will need to get some sort of fluid circulation from the capsule of the joint, hence the swelling and tenderness in the joint capsule. The inflammatory process may appear as if there is infection when there is only dehydration.

joint surfaces. It seems that they cater to the lines of force and pressure that the joints have to endure.

Unfortunately, the repair process seems to produce a deviation of the joints. To avoid such disfigurement, one should take the initial pain very seriously and give strict attention to daily intake of water. This pain should be recognised as a sign of local dehydration. If it does not disappear after a few days of water intake and repeated gentle bending of the joints to bring more circulation to the area, one should then consult a professional practitioner of medicine.

You have nothing to lose and everything to gain by recognising the pain and the non-infectious inflammation of a rheumatoid joint as a thirst signal in your body. You are probably showing other signals for water shortage in your body, but this particular site is indicating predisposition to a more severe local damage.

If we understand the body to have difficulty in recognising its thirst state, it is possible that this lower state of alertness is also inheritable by a child. It is possible that dehydration in a rapidly growing child might also indicate its presence by the pain felt in the joints, as well as in heartburn. The mode of signal production that would denote thirst might naturally be the same in the young as in older people. It is therefore recommended that juvenile arthritis should also be treated with an increase in daily water intake.

As you can see, Dr Laurence Malone, whose letter is published on page 48, is an experienced medical doctor and an educator. His observations on the effect of water on rheumatoid joint pains in himself show that our other colleagues in the medical profession should begin to notice the medicinal values of water in disease prevention.

Low back pain

It should be appreciated that the spinal joints - intervertebral joints and their disc structures - are dependent on different hydraulic properties of water stored in the disc core, as well as in the end plate cartilage covering the flat surfaces of the spinal vertebrae. In spinal vertebral joints, water is not only a lubricant for the contact surfaces, it is held in the disc core within the intervertebral space and supports the compression weight of the upper part of the body. *Fully*

Dean for Academic Affairs
Laurence A. Malone MD PhD.

(216) 543-8977
12-18-93

The Learning Center

Global Health Solutions, Inc.,
P.O. Box 3189
Falls Church, Va.22043

Attn: The Honorable F. Batmanghelid, M.D.

Gentlemen:

At 82 years of age I am still in fair shape and only
regret I did not have the superb advice of Dr. Batmanghelid and
that of his books "Your Body's Many Cries for Water" and "Low
Back Pain".

Dr. Batman's reasoning is incisive, his medical knowledge
indeed sparkles with wit and brilliant logic. His books are now a
treasured possession in my library. I have used his advice for
the painful arthritis I have in my hands and back and within two
weeks, I have experienced considerable reduction of pain. I sleep
better, I have more strength, with greater coordination and relaxation.
I see life from a different point of view, where everything seems
easier for me to do.

Dr. Batman's books are full of common sense and truthful
medical advice. His suggested treatment of disease goes to the roots,
the cause of it and anyone who is fortunate enough to read them won't
be disappointed with their purchase.

Respectfully,

Laurence A. Malone.

"A Tutorial Learning Center For College Sciences"
(Licensed By The State of Ohio)

8225 East Washington Street   Chagrin Falls, Ohio 44023

75 per cent of the weight of the upper part of the body is supported by the water volume that is stored in the disc core; 25 per cent is supported by the fibrous materials around the disc (see Figure 8 overleaf). In all joints, water acts as a lubricating agent and it bears the force produced by weight or the tension produced by muscle action on the joint.

In most of these joints, the establishment of an intermittent vacuum promotes a silent water circulation into the joint, only for it to be squeezed out by pressure borne as a result of joint activity. To prevent back pain, one needs to drink sufficient water and do a series of special exercises to create an intermittent vacuum to draw water into the disc space. These exercises will also reduce the spasm in the back muscles that, in the vast majority of people, is the main cause of lower back pain. One also needs to adopt correct postures.

The subject of back pain and its relationship to water is so important that I have dealt with it in a special book, *How to Deal With Back Pain and Rheumatoid Joint Pain,* and a complementary video, *How To Deal With Back Pain.* If you get back pain and in particular sciatic pain, you will benefit by reading the book and seeing the video. In a majority of cases sciatic pain can be totally relieved within half an hour when the special movements that produce an intermittent vacuum in the disc spaces – as shown in the book and video – are performed.

Neck pain

Bad posture, keeping the head bent for long periods when writing, working at a low bench, 'freeze position' while at the computer for many hours, a bad pillow or too many pillows can be contributory factors in the production of neck pain, or even the displacement of the intervertebral discs in the neck. Neck movement is essential for the establishment of adequate fluid circulation within the disc spaces in the neck. The weight of the head forces water out of the discs over a period of time. To bring back the same water, the force of vacuum has to be created within the same disc space. This can only be done if the head and neck are moved adequately backward.

A simple process in less severe cases of neck pain from disc

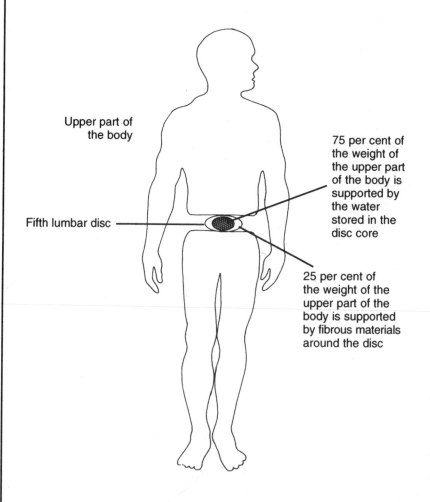

The importance of the fifth lumbar disc

Upper part of the body

Fifth lumbar disc

75 per cent of the weight of the upper part of the body is supported by the water stored in the disc core

25 per cent of the weight of the upper part of the body is supported by fibrous materials around the disc

Figure 8: A schematic model showing the importance of water to the disc core. It provides the essential hydraulic support for the weight-bearing qualities of an intervertebral disc. Once dehydration sets in, all the parts of the body begin to suffer. The intervertebral discs and their joints are first in line. The fifth lumbar disc is affected in 95 per cent of cases.

displacement would be slowly and *repeatedly* bending the head and neck backward, as much as they will bend, keeping the neck extended for 30 seconds at a time. This extension enhances the force of vacuum and brings water into the disc spaces. At the same time, because of their front attachment to the spinal ligament, all of the discs will be retracted back into their normal spaces between the vertebrae and away from the nerve roots in the neck.

Another simple procedure to correct this problem is lying on one's back on the very edge of the bed with the head hanging back and down. This posture permits the weight of the head to stretch the non-weight-bearing neck and bend it backward. A few moments of total relaxation in this position will ease the tension in the neck. This is a good posture to generate a type of vacuum in the disc spaces in the neck. After gently bending the head backward so that you can see the floor, raise the head until you see the wall beyond your feet. This procedure may be effective in creating an intermittent vacuum in the vertebral spaces between any two vertebrae. The vacuum draws water into the disc spaces and spreads it to all parts in the neck joints and lubricates their movements. This water is needed for the disc core to re-expand to its natural size, jacking up and separating one vertebra from the other. You could now bend the head from one side to the other. Try to look at the wall and floor of the room, first one side and then the other side. People who begin to suffer from neck 'arthritis', or disc displacement in the neck, may wish to test this simple procedure to improve the mobility of their neck joints.

Anginal pain

For more information read the section on cholesterol. In brief and to address the dehydration-produced pains of the body together, anginal pain means water shortage in the body. The common factor in all the conditions labelled as different diseases of the heart and the lungs is an established dehydration.

Take a look at Mr Samuel Liguori's and Loretta Johnson's letters, published by their kind permission (among the testimonials in the section on cholesterol, pages 86 and 88). Mr Liguori's anginal pain disappeared when he started to increase his water intake. He also had suffered from hiatus hernia and that too started to clear up. Given time, it will clear up completely. You willk see from Loretta Johnson's letter that, even at the young-at-heart age of 90, anginal pain can be treated with water, to the extent that she does not need any medication for her heart pains.

Headaches

In my personal experience, migraine headaches seem to be brought about by dehydration; excess bed covers that will not permit the body to regulate its temperature during sleep; alcoholic beverages (hangover) initiating a process of cellular dehydration, particularly in the brain; dietary or allergic triggers for histamine release; excess environmental heat without water intake. Basically, migraine seems to be an indicator of critical body temperature regulation at times of 'heat stress'. Dehydration plays a major role in the precipitation of migraine headaches.

The most prudent way of dealing with migraine is its prevention by the regular intake of water. Once migraine breaks the pain barriers, a cascade of chemical reactions will stop the body from further activity. At this time, one has to take pain-relieving medications with copious water. Sufficient cold or iced water may by itself be able to cool the body (also the brain) from inside, and promote closing of the vascular system everywhere. Excess dilation of the peripheral vessels might well be the basic cause of migraine headache.

Mrs Mavis Butler, a touring Australian Adventist missionary in Silang in the Philippines, has an interesting history. She has for many years suffered from migraine headaches. She would at times be so incapacitated as to become bed-ridden. She came across this book when she was in Silang and started to increase her water intake. She wrote to tell me that she has so improved that she now wants to shout it from the house tops.

Mrs Butler's long letter is reprinted on the following pages. Hers is another of those human stories that make one wonder how it is possible that we were so ignorant of the importance of water to health that people could suffer from its lack in the body, to the point of wishing to die.

P O Box 1619, Innisfail 4860
North Queensland, Australia
January 23, 1995

Dear Dr. Batmanghelidj:
For many years I suffered with headaches. I consulted doctors, neurologists, chiropractors and spent hundreds of dollars for head-scans and X-rays, all to no avail. At times only my faith in God kept me from wanting to die, as I lie prone on my bed for days on end in pain.

No medication would ever stop the pain, it would just seem to run its course and then stop. I could never make any connection between my diet and the headaches, and the only pattern they seemed to follow was to always start a couple of hours after a meal.

Then one day a friend told me that he thought my headaches were caused because I never drank enough water. While I knew I didn't actually drink much water, I thought my herbal tea with fruit juices together with lots of fruits amply supplied my liquid requirements. Just three weeks later I was leafing through a health magazine when an advertisement for your book, 'Your Body's Many Cries for Water', just seemed to leap out at my eyes. I bought the magazine and sent for the book.

When it came, I eagerly read and re-read it to learn this new concept about water, and as I saw the errors in my drinking habits I quickly set about to righting them. Can anyone, without experiencing it for themselves, really understand what it is like to have usually pain-filled days changed to wonderful painless days when you can do the things you want to do, instead of being 'down with a headache?'. Oh, such a blessing for which I thank God continually.

It has taken months to properly hydrate my body, but now a headache is a now-and-again event instead of the norm. I thank a loving and caring God for leading me step by step to this wonderful truth. He no doubt tried to lead me a lot earlier, but I was too blind to see. I thank you, doctor, for your great work and perseverance in bringing this truth to the people.

I lecture to adults at night classes on 'Better Food and Eating Habits' and I quickly gave one of my sessions entirely to the body's need for water. I have been able to help many people to better health and much less pain in their lives, with this knowledge. A friend told me he was going into hospital in a few days time for stomach and ulcer treatment. I begged him to cancel this and try the water treatment you recommended.

He somewhat reluctantly did and was amazed and thankful to find his pains stop and in time, to know that the ulcer had healed, all without medication.

Please let me offer my grateful thanks again and pray that the Lord will bless and guide you and your staff as you work for the better health of humanity.
Sincerely,

(Mrs) Mavis Butler

CHAPTER 5

Stress and depression

'The reasonable man adapts himself to the world:
the unreasonable one persists in trying to adapt
the world to himself. Therefore all progress
depends on the unreasonable man.'
George Bernard Shaw

A state of depression is said to exist when the brain, in confronting a stressful emotional problem, finds it difficult to cope with other attention-demanding actions at the same time. This phenomenon can become so all-absorbing as to incapacitate the person. In the long run, such a stressful drain on brain activity can produce different manifestations that are labelled according to the person's outward behaviour pattern.

Ten million Americans are said to be suffering from one form or another of such serious conditions. Infinitely greater numbers are experiencing, or will at one time or another experience, the milder forms of depression. In Britain, it is estimated that : 'At any given point in time, about 20 per cent of the population will have some depressive symptoms, not just sadness . . .' (MIND).

Some form of depression is a natural phenomenon in the process of development and progress of any individual. It is in these states of consuming mental activity that characters are developed and the inner mettle of the individual is forged. Naturally, coping with different aspects of one's negative feelings is part and parcel of the process. Almost always, the state of depression is a passing phenomenon if love, care, and empathy are available to nudge the individual in the direction of a resolution of negative inner thoughts.

Unfortunately, some people will not be able to cope with the fear, anxiety and anger associated with depression. In seeking professional help, they are given some form of medication. At the onset of chemical treatment of depression, the medications were less harmful. Today, they are very powerful and sometimes dangerous. Some forms of treatment will strip away the emotional ability to feel for themselves, as well as for others. Some of these medications can destroy empathy and fix a negative idea in particularly vulnerable persons. They may more easily become suicidal, as well as antisocial and homicidal.

What I am setting out to explain in this chapter is the reason for inefficiency of the physiology associated with stress and depression. What I propose is the way to increase the efficiency of brain power to cope with extremely severe emotional stress and its outward manifestations of depression. I have experienced, and have observed in many others, all of the positive aspects to what I am proposing.

Pathology that is seen to be associated with social stresses – fear, anxiety, insecurity, persistent emotional and matrimonial problems and the establishment of depression – is the result of water deficiency to the point that the water requirement of brain tissue is affected. The brain uses electrical energy that is generated by the water drive of the energy-generating pumps. With dehydration, the level of energy generation in the brain is decreased. Many functions of the brain that depend on this type of energy become inefficient. We recognise this inadequacy of function and call it *depression*. This depressive state caused by dehydration can lead to *chronic fatigue syndrome*. This condition is a label put on a series of advanced physiological problems that are seen to be associated with stress.

If we understand the events that take place in stress, we will also understand chronic fatigue syndrome. In any case, after a period of time of correcting for dehydration and its metabolic complications, chronic fatigue syndrome will improve beyond recognition. The following pages define the physiological events and the possible metabolic over-rides that can lead to depletion of certain body reserves that may be the basic problem in chronic fatigue syndrome.

Initially silent compensation mechanisms

When the body becomes dehydrated, the physiological processes that will be established are the same ones that occur when coping with stress. Dehydration equals stress and, once stress is established, there is an associated mobilisation of primary materials from body stores. This process will mop up some of the water reserves of the body. Consequently, dehydration causes stress, and stress will cause further dehydration.

In stress, several hormonal overrides become operative. The body assumes a crisis situation and will begin to mobilise for a fight or flight response. The body does not seem to recognise the social transformation of humans. It assesses all situations of stress as though a fight or flight stance has to be maintained, even with those stresses associated with work in an office. Several strong hormones become secreted and will remain triggered until the body gets out of its stressful circumstances. These hormones are mainly *endorphins, cortisone release factor, prolactin, vasopressin,* and *renin-angiotensin.*

Endorphins, cortisone, prolactin and vasopressin

Endorphins prepare the body to endure hardship and injury until it gets out of danger. They also raise the pain threshold. With an injury that would have caused pain at a lower level, with the 'umbrella' of endorphins, the body will be able to continue with its task. Because of childbirth and monthly menstruation, women seem to access this hormone much more readily. *They generally have a greater ability to withstand pain and stress.*

Cortisone will initiate the demobilisation of stored energies and raw materials. Fat is broken down into fatty acids to be converted into energy. Some proteins are once again broken down into the basic amino acids for the formation of extra neurotransmitters, new proteins, and some special amino acids to be burned by the muscles. During pregnancy and at the time of feeding milk to the child, this hormone and its 'associates' will mobilise a uniform flow of primary materials for the purpose of offspring development. If the action of cortisone continues for long, soon there will be some selective depletion from the amino acid reserves of the body.

Under the influence of cortisone, the body continues to 'feed off itself'. The effect of cortisone is designed to provide emergency raw materials for the production of most essential primary proteins and neurotransmitters to get the body 'over the hump'. It is not designed for the continued breakdown of materials employed in maintenance of the structural integrity of the body. It is this phenomenon that produces the damage associated with stress, if the stressor maintains its unabated influence.

Prolactin will make sure that the lactating mother will continue to produce milk. All species have it. Prolactin will prime the gland cells in the breast to continue with milk production even if there is

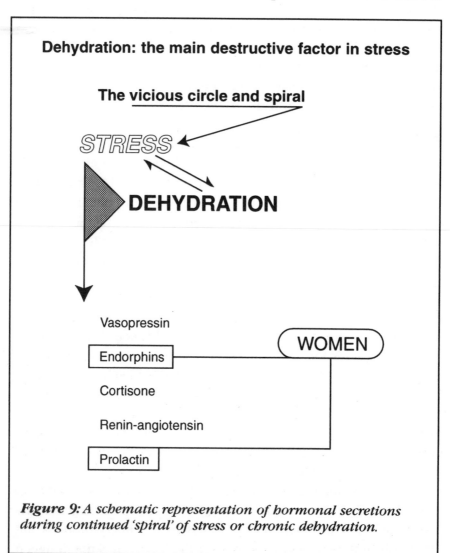

Figure 9: *A schematic representation of hormonal secretions during continued 'spiral' of stress or chronic dehydration.*

dehydration or stress that will cause dehydration. It will prime the gland cells to regenerate and increase in quantity.

We should remember that, although we concentrate on the solid composition of the milk, it is its water content that is of primary importance to the growing foetus. Every time a cell gives rise to a daughter cell, 75 per cent or more of its volume has to be filled with water. In short, growth depends on the availability of water. When water is brought to the area, the cells will be able to access its other dissolved contents. This hormone is also made in the placenta and stored in the amniotic fluid surrounding the foetus. In short, this hormone has a mammotrophic action. It makes the breast glands and their ducts grow. Growth hormone has much similarity to prolactin. They have similar actions, except that prolactin mainly targets the organs of reproduction.

It has been shown in mice that increased prolactin production will cause mammary tumours. In 1987, I proposed in my guest lecture address to a select international group of cancer researchers that chronic dehydration in the human body is a primary causative factor in the production of tumours. The relationship between stress, age-dependent chronic dehydration, persistent prolactin secretion, and cancer transformation of the glandular tissue in the breast should not be overlooked. A regular adjustment to the daily water intake in women – particularly when confronting stresses of everyday life – will at the very least serve as a preventive measure against possible development of stress-induced breast cancer in the age group of women predisposed to this problem and of prostate cancer in men.

Vasopressin regulates the selective flow of water into some cells of the body. It also causes a constriction of the capillaries it activates. As its name implies, it causes vaso-constriction. It is produced in the pituitary gland and secreted into the circulation. While it may constrict blood vessels, some vital cells possess receiving points (receptors) for this hormone. Depending on the hierarchy of their importance, some cells seem to possess more vasopressin receptors than others.

The cell membrane – the protective covering of cell architecture – is naturally designed in two layers. Tuning-fork-like solid hydrocarbon 'bricks' are held together by the adhesive property of water (see

Water filtration through cell membranes

A single nerve cell

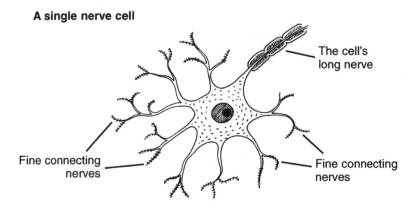

The cell's
long nerve

Fine connecting
nerves

Fine connecting
nerves

A microscopic segment of nerve cell membrane

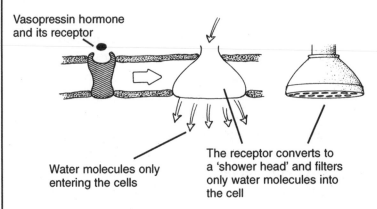

Vasopressin hormone
and its receptor

Water molecules only
entering the cells

The receptor converts to
a 'shower head' and filters
only water molecules into
the cell

Figure 10: *A schematic model of a nerve cell, its bilayer membrane, and the vasopressin receptor that converts into a 'shower head' structure and enables the filtered water from the serum to enter the cells that have the receptor. Vasopressin also produces vasoconstriction, which puts a squeeze on the blood volume to produce the pressure for water filtration - reverse osmosis.*

Figure 14, page 80). In between the two layers there is a connecting passageway where enzymes travel, selectively react together, and cause a desired action within the cell. This waterway works very much like a moat or 'beltway', except that it is a water-filled beltway and everything has to float in it.

When there is sufficient water to fill all the spaces, the moat gets filled and water will also get into the cell. There may come a time when the rate of water flow into the cell may not be sufficient, and some of the cell functions may become affected. To safeguard against such a potentially catastrophic situation, nature has designed a magnificent mechanism for the creation of water filters through the membrane. When vasopressin hormone reaches the cell membrane and fuses with its specially designed receptor, the receptor converts to a 'shower head' structure and makes possible filtration of water only through its holes.

The important cells manufacture the vasopressin receptor in greater quantity. Vasopressin is one of the hormones involved in the rationing and distribution of water according to a priority plan when there is dehydration. Nerve cells seem to exercise their priority by manufacturing more vasopressin receptors than other tissue cells. They need to keep the waterways in their nerves fully functional. To make sure the water can pass through these tiny holes (which only allow the passage of one water molecule at a time), vasopressin also has the property of causing vasoconstriction and putting a squeeze on the fluid volume in the region.

Thus, the hypertensive property of the neurotransmitter vaso-pressin, better known as a hormone, is needed to bring about a steady filtration of water into the cells, only when the free flow and direct diffusion of water through the cell membrane is not enough. Figure 10 explains this mechanism. For more information on the cell membrane, read the section on cholesterol.

Alcohol

Alcohol will suppress the secretion of vasopressin from the pituitary gland. Lack of vasopressin in circulation will translate to general dehydration of the body even in the brain cells. Now, a previously

The transport system in the nerves

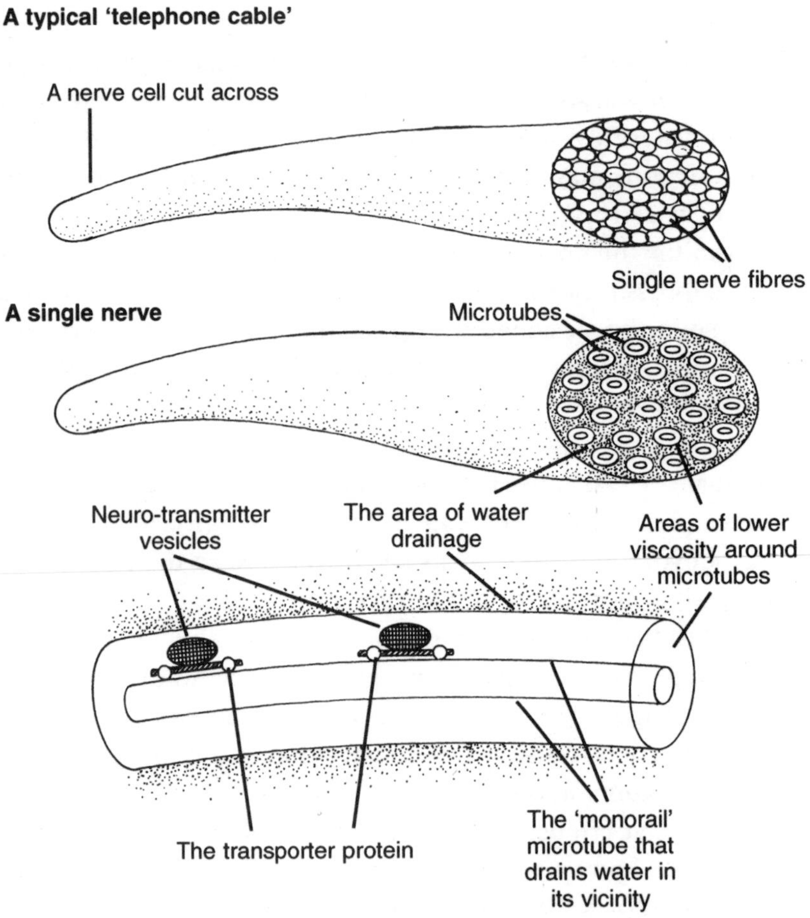

A typical 'telephone cable'

A nerve cell cut across

Single nerve fibres

A single nerve

Microtubes

Neuro-transmitter vesicles

The area of water drainage

Areas of lower viscosity around microtubes

The transporter protein

The 'monorail' microtube that drains water in its vicinity

Figure 11: A schematic model (also shown in Figure 3) to demonstrate the mechanism of 'float' transport system within lesser viscosity microstream flow systems that become established around 'monorail' type of structures called microtubules – particularly along the length of nerves.

slight and easier-to-adjust-to dehydration will translate to a very severe drought in the 'sensitive cells' of the brain. To cope with this stress, more of the various hormones are secreted, including the body's own addictive *endorphins*.

Thus, prolonged use of alcohol may be instrumental in promoting addictive tendencies to endorphin secretion in the body, triggering the secretion of excess endorphins. Women, because of their natural tendency to increase endorphin production to cope with childbirth and their monthly menstruation, seem to become addicted to alcohol more readily than men. It seems that women become addicted to alcohol in about three years, compared to men who may become compulsive drinkers in about seven years.

Figures 10 and 11 explain some of the factors possibly contributing to the development of chronic fatigue syndrome during an expanding chronic dehydration. It can occur from the regular intake of caffeine-containing and alcoholic beverages in place of water. The vasopressin receptor is naturally designed to keep the *waterways* in the nerve systems fully *topped-up*. Naturally, in dehydration of the nerve system, the energy and volition to do new work is drastically reduced.

Renin-angiotensin system

Renin-angiotensin (RA) system activity (see Figure 12 overleaf) is a subordinate mechanism to histamine activation in the brain. The RA system is also recognised to be very strongly active in the kidneys. This system is activated when the body's fluid volume is diminished. It is activated to retain water, and to do so, it also promotes the absorption of more salt. In either water or sodium depletion of the body, the RA system becomes very active.

Until the water and sodium content of the body reach a preset level, the RA system also brings about the tightening of the capillary bed and the vascular system. It is designed to do this so there is no 'slack' and empty space in the circulation system. This tightening can reach such a level that it becomes measurable, and at which point it is called *hypertension*. You think a reading of 200 points is high? I have seen the blood pressure of a man without prior history of hypertension reach a level of 300 millimetres of mercury, *300 points*, when he was arrested and taken to one of the Iranian political prisons to be shot.

The reason for this tightening of the blood vessels during stress is simple to understand. The body is a highly integrated and efficient complex multi-system. When there is stress, some of the available

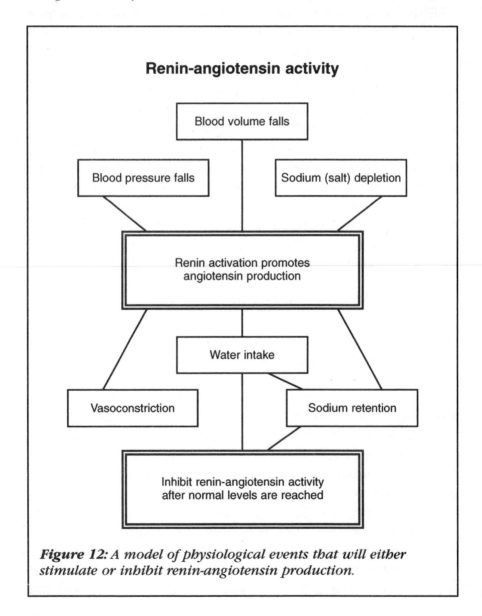

Figure 12: *A model of physiological events that will either stimulate or inhibit renin-angiotensin production.*

water is used for the breakdown of stored materials like proteins, starch (glycogen) and fat. To compensate for the lost water and to put the system into a squeeze, the RA system will also co-ordinate work with vasopressin and other hormones. The kidneys are the main site of RA system activity.

The kidneys are responsible for urine production and excretion of excess hydrogen, potassium, sodium, and waste materials. All of these functions have to be maintained proportionate to sufficient availability of water to be used to make urine. True, the kidneys have the ability to concentrate the urine. However, this ability is not to be used to its extreme at all times, or it will eventually produce kidney damage.

The RA system is the pivotal mechanism for the restoration of fluid volume in the body. It is one of the subordinate mechanisms to histamine activity for water intake. It regulates the vascular bed to adjust for the fluid content of the circulation system. Its activity is decreased by the presence of more salt and water to fill the fluid capacity of the vascular bed. In the kidneys, it senses the fluid flow and the filtration pressure for its urine-making system. If the filtration pressure is not adequate for urine filtration and secretion, the RA system will tighten the blood vessels in this organ.

When the kidneys are damaged and urine production is insufficient, the RA system is more active. It promotes more salt intake and induces more thirst. Kidney damage may be the consequence of long-term dehydration and salt depletion that had triggered the RA system activity in the first place. But we have not in the past recognised the significance of the vascular tightening (essential hypertension) as an indicator of body's fluid loss. Now, insufficient fluid balance in the body may have to be considered as the primary factor in some cases of renal damage to the point of needing kidney replacement. Once the RA system is turned fully ON, it continues its expanding pace until a natural switching system turns it off. The components of the natural OFF switch are *WATER AND SOME SALT in that order* until the measurable vascular tightening indicates a normal range.

The salivary glands seem to have the ability to sense salt shortage in the body. When there is sodium shortage, they seem to produce substances called *kinins*. Kinins promote added blood circulation and increased saliva formation in the *salivary glands*. This increased saliva formation (possibly to the extent that it would flow out of the mouth) serves two purposes: it lubricates the mouth during food intake in a dehydrated state of the body and its alkaline consistency and copious flow will assist in food breakdown and its eventual evacuation from the stomach. Within the integrated systems of the human body, kinins of the salivary gland seem also to trigger activation of the RA system that will begin to influence all parts of the body.

Thus, sodium (salt) shortage in the body (also contributing to a devastating water shortage outside cells) could initiate a series of events that would ultimately produce essential hypertension and chronic pains in humans. The relationship of the salivary kinins to sodium depletion (salt depletion causes body water content loss) and ample saliva production, even if the body is fairly dehydrated, is a paradox in the design of the human body. It exposes the gross error of considering the 'dry mouth' as the sole indicator of water shortage in humans! Because of this basic error, the practice of medicine and scientific research are light years off course. Much backtracking and revision to the already adopted views will be unavoidable.

What happens if we drink tea, coffee, or colas in place of water? Natural stimulants in coffee and tea are larger quantities of caffeine and lesser amounts of theophylline (theafelin). These are central nervous system stimulants. At the same time, *they are dehydrating agents because of their strong diuretic action on the kidneys.* One cup of coffee contains about 85 milligrams of caffeine, and one cup of tea about 50 milligrams of caffeine. Colas contain about 50 milligrams of caffeine, part of which is added to standardise the recipe when extracting the active substances from the nuts of *cola accuminata.*

These central nervous system stimulants liberate energy from the ATP storage pool and convert ATP to its burnt stage of cyclic AMP in the cells – at certain levels, a strong inhibitory agent. They also release energy from liberation of calcium from its stored form in the cells. Thus, caffeine seems to act in an energy releasing capacity in the body. We all know about this final effect of caffeine; what we should also know is its override effect when the body does not wish to release energy for a certain action. In this way, the action of some hormones and transmitters will not be limited at a later time because of a possible lower level of stored energy. Caffeine will cause an override effect *until a lower level of energy storage is reached.* Cola drinks have exactly the same effect.

The effect of caffeine may at some times be considered desirable, *but constant substituting of caffeine-containing drinks for water will deprive the body of its full capacity for the formation of hydroelectric energy.* Excess caffeine will also deplete the ATP-stored energy in the brain and the body – a possible contributing factor for shorter attention span in the younger, cola-consuming generation, or chronic fatigue syndrome as a result of excess coffee consumption in later life. Excess caffeine intake will eventually exhaust the heart muscle because of its over-stimulation.

Recently, in some experimental models, it has been shown that caffeine inhibits a most important enzyme system, PDE (phospho-di-esterase), that is involved in the process of learning and memory development. In reported experiments, caffeine impaired vision and memory components of learning ability in the species involved in the experiment.

You must now realise why people with Alzheimer's disease and children with a learning disability should not drink anything other than water. Caffeine-containing beverages should definitely NOT be consumed.

Let us now connect all the information given in this chapter with two different but related problems – hypertension and cholesterol formation – both leading to heart problems.

The operating mechanism for adaptation to dehydration, which will climax into vasoconstriction, is the same as mentioned for stress. Namely, the continued actions of vasopressin and the RA system are responsible for establishing the necessary adaptation to drought. They close a number of open capillaries in the vascular bed and increase the pressure in the rest to squeeze water through the membranes into the cells in 'priority organs'. Do not forget this simple truth: dehydration is the number one stressor of the human body – or *any* living matter.

October 20, 1995

Dr. F. Batmanghelidj
Global Health Solutions Inc.
P.O. Box 3189
Fairfax, VA 22043

Dear Dr. Batmanghelidj:

I am a person with M.S. I have been using the greatest health discovery in history program (drink 2qts. of water daily, no caffeine and adding some salt as seasoning) for four weeks. I can confidently state that I am thrilled with the incredible results. Previously, I had been plagued by bad swelling of my legs for years. Within two weeks the swelling had gone down 90 percent.

As an M.S. client, I am also grateful to be free of my caffeine and sugar roller coaster that I was on. I am excited about my increased and consistent energy which lasts all day and into the evening. I am without the downside of exhaustion which followed the caffeine bursts. I was chained to that roller coaster which only made my fatigue spells during the day so much more severe. Now that I am free from that cycle, I also notice that I am calmer, less anxious and more productive. Also, I am more optimistic about things in general, more able to give of myself to others and more attentive to the natural rhythms of my body that I previously masked chemically by caffeine.

Truly your discovery has given me back a large portion of my life.

Sincerely,

John Kuna
RD1
Box 1488
Nicholson, Pa. 18446

P.S   I would be more than happy to speak with anyone who has an interest in what I have found out.

CHAPTER 6

High blood pressure

*'Physicians think they are doing
something for you by labelling
what you have as a disease.'*
Immanuel Kant

High blood pressure (essential hypertension) is the result of an adaptive process to a gross body water deficiency.

The vessels of the body have been designed to cope with fluctuation of their blood volume and tissue requirements by opening and closing different vessels. When the body's total fluid volume is decreased, the main vessels also have to decrease their aperture (close their lumina), otherwise there would not be enough fluid to fill all the space allocated to blood volume in the design of that particular body. Failing a capacity adjustment to the 'water volume' by the blood vessels, gases would separate from the blood and fill the space, causing 'gas locks'. This property of lumen regulation for fluid circulation is a most advanced design within the principle of hydraulics and after which the blood circulation of the body is modelled.

Shunting of blood circulation is a normal routine. When we eat, most of the circulation is directed into the intestinal tract by closing some capillary circulation elsewhere. When we eat, more capillaries are opened in the gastrointestinal tract and fewer are open in the major muscle systems. Only areas where activity places a more urgent demand on the circulatory systems will be kept fully open for the passage of blood. In other words, it is the blood-holding capacity of the capillary bed that determines the direction and rate of flow to any site at a given time.

This process is naturally designed to cope with any priority work without the burden of maintaining an excess fluid volume in the body. When the act of digestion has taken place and less blood is needed in the gastrointestinal region, circulation to other areas will

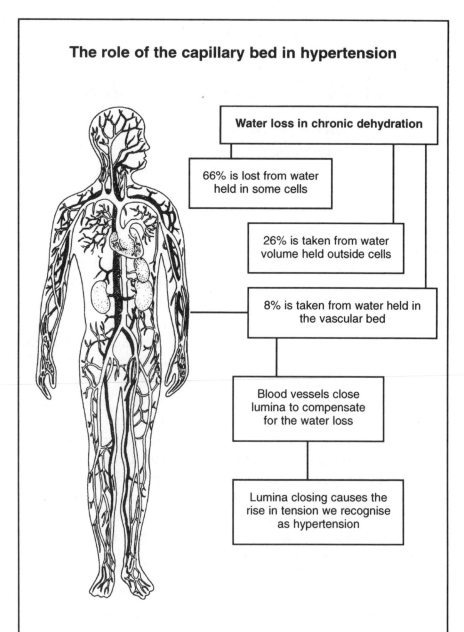

The role of the capillary bed in hypertension

Water loss in chronic dehydration

66% is lost from water held in some cells

26% is taken from water volume held outside cells

8% is taken from water held in the vascular bed

Blood vessels close lumina to compensate for the water loss

Lumina closing causes the rise in tension we recognise as hypertension

Figure 13: The vascular system all over the body adapts to the blood volume loss by selective closing of its lumina. A major cause of blood volume loss is the loss of body water or its under-supply through losing thirst sensation.

open more easily. In a most indirect way, this is why we feel less active immediately after a meal and ready for action after some time has passed. In short, there is a mechanism for establishment of priority for circulating blood to any given area – some capillaries open and some others close. The order is predetermined according to a scale of importance of function. The brain, lungs, liver, kidneys, and glands take priority over muscles, bones, and skin in blood distribution *unless* a different priority is programmed into the system. This will happen if a continued demand on any part of the body influences the extent of blood circulation to the area, such as muscle development through regular exercise.

Water shortage: potentials for hypertension

When we do not drink enough water to serve all the needs of the body, some cells become dehydrated and lose some of their water to the circulation. Capillary beds in some areas will have to close so that some of the slack in capacity is adjusted for. *In water shortage and body drought, 66 per cent is taken from the water volume normally held inside the cells; 26 per cent is taken from the volume held outside the cells; and 8 per cent is taken from blood volume* (see Figure 13). There is no alternative for the blood vessels other than closing their lumina to cope with the loss in blood volume. The process begins by closing some capillaries in less active areas. The deficient quantity must come either from outside or be taken from another part of the body.

It is the extent of capillary bed activity throughout the body that will ultimately determine the volume of circulating blood. The more the muscles are exercised, the more their capillaries will open and hold a greater volume of blood within the circulation reserves. *This is the reason why exercise is a very important component for physiological adjustments in those suffering from hypertension.* This is one aspect to the physiology of hypertension. The capillary bed must remain open and full and offer no resistance to blood circulation. When the capillary bed is closed and offers resistance, only an increased force behind the circulating blood will ensure the passage of some fluids through the system.

Another reason why the capillary bed may become selectively closed is shortage of water in the body. *Basically, water we drink will ultimately have to get into the cells - water regulates the volume of a cell from inside. Salt regulates the amount of water that is held outside the cells - the ocean around the cell.* There is a very delicate balancing process in the design of the body in the way it maintains its composition of blood at the expense of fluctuating the water content in some cells of the body.

When there is a shortage of water, some cells will go without a portion of their normal needs and others will get a predetermined rationed amount to maintain function (as explained, the mechanism involves water filtration through the cell membrane). However, blood will normally retain the consistency of its composition. It must do so in order to keep the normal composition of elements reaching the vital centres.

This is where the solutes paradigm is inadequate and goes wrong. It bases all assessments and evaluations of body functions on the solids content of blood. It does not recognise the comparative dehydration of some other parts of the body. All blood tests can appear normal and yet the small capillaries of the heart and the brain may be closed and cause some of the cells of these organs a gradual damage from increasing dehydration over a long period of time. When you read the section on cholesterol formation, this statement will become more clear.

When we lose thirst sensation (or do not recognise other signals of dehydration) and drink less water than the daily requirement, the shutting down of some vascular beds is the only natural alternative to keep the rest of the blood vessels full. The question is, how long can we go on like this? The answer is, long enough to ultimately become very ill and die. Unless we get wise to the paradigm shift, and professionally and generally begin to recognise the problems associated with water metabolism disturbance in the human body and its variety of thirst signals, *chronic dehydration will continue to take its toll on both our bodies and our society!*

Essential hypertension should primarily be treated with an increase in daily water intake. The present way of treating hypertension is wrong to the point of *scientific absurdity.* The body is trying to retain its water volume, and we say to the design of nature in us: 'No, you do not understand – you must take diuretics and get rid of water!' It so happens that, if we do not drink sufficient water, the only other way the body has to secure water is through the mechanism of keeping sodium in the body. The RA system is directly involved. Only when sodium is retained will water remain in the extra-cellular fluid compartment. From this compartment, through the mechanism of shower-head production, water will be forced into some of the cells with 'priority' status. *Thus, keeping sodium in the body is a last resort way of retaining some water for its 'shower-head' filtered use.*

There is a sensitivity of design attached to sodium retention in the body. To assume this to be the cause of hypertension is inaccurate and stems from insufficient knowledge of the water regulatory mechanisms in the human body. When diuretics are given to get rid of the sodium, the body becomes more dehydrated. The dry mouth level of dehydration is reached and water is taken to compensate. Diuretics maintain the body at an expanding level of deficit water management. They do not cure hypertension; they make the body more determined for salt and water absorption, but never enough to correct the problem. That is why, after a while, diuretics are not enough and supplemental medications will be forced on the patient.

Another problem in assessment of hypertension is its means of measurement. *Anxiety associated with having hypertension will automatically affect the person at examination time.* Readings of the instruments may not reflect the true, natural and normal blood pressure. An inexperienced or hasty medical practitioner, more in fear of litigation than mindful of accuracy of judgement, might assume the patient to have hypertension, whereas the person might only have an instant of 'clinic anxiety', thus causing a higher reading of the instrument. One other very important but less-known problem with the mechanism of reading blood pressure is the process of inflating the cuff well above the systolic reading, and then letting the air out until the pulse is heard.

Every large (and possibly small) artery has a companion nerve that is there to monitor the flow of blood through the vessel. With the loss of pressure beyond the cuff that is now inflated to very high levels, the process of 'pressure' opening of the obstruction in the arteries will be triggered. By the time the pressure in the cuff is lowered to read the pulsation level, the recording of an artificially induced higher blood pressure will have become unavoidable. Unfortunately, the measurement of hypertension is so arbitrary (and based on the diastolic level) that in this litigious society a minor error in assessment may label a person hypertensive. This is when all the fun and games begin!

Water by itself is the best natural diuretic. If people who have hypertension, and produce adequate urine, increase their daily water intake, they will not need to take diuretics. If prolonged 'hypertension producing dehydration' has also caused heart failure complications, water intake should be increased gradually. In this way, one makes sure that fluid collection in the body is not excessive or unmanageable.

The mechanism of sodium retention in these people is in overdrive mode. When water intake is increased gradually and more urine is being produced, the oedema fluid (swelling) that is full of toxic substances will be flushed out, and the heart will regain its strength.

The following four letters are presented with the kind permission of their authors, who wished to share their welcome experiences with the readers of this book. The first is from Marjori Ramsay, a lady in her early eighties.

Dear Dr Batmanghelidj
November 22, 1993

I have just ordered another copy of your book on water, having given a son my first copy. I tell everybody about it and my experiences. Perhaps you would be interested.

My first son Charles, 58, who lives with me, is deaf and autistic. I take him three or four days a week to a facility for the handicapped. They had been taking his blood pressure there and notified me that the doctor said he should go on medication - his BP was 140-160/100-104. I had just received your book and asked the

M.D. to let me experiment for two weeks. Reluctantly he agreed, but warned me it was very dangerous.

I kept Charles home and used the water routine, also adding a little magnesium and potassium.

Two weeks later the nurse took his BP and it was 106/80. She said: 'The doctor will be in shortly'- evidently the M.D. didn't believe her and he checked it himself and had to admit it was so. He didn't ask me what I did, so I did not tell him about water, but if the BP continues as it is, I will tell him.

I went on the water routine too without any particular problem in mind, but noticed that in about 10 days my tendency to get dizzy if I moved my head quickly had disappeared. I also had been unable to lower my head to lie flat at nights and had to have several pillows. Now I am much better, and have had only one spell in over a month: I am 82 years of age.

Thank you for the work you are doing - it is much needed. More power to you.

Marjori Ramsay

If you can find out why this particular doctor was not interested in discovering how Charles's mother brought his blood pressure back to normal, you will then realise why we have a health care crisis on our hands!

The writer of the second letter is Michael Peck. He has, in the past, been involved in an administrative capacity with the Foundation for the Simple in Medicine, which I helped to establish. The foundation is a medical research ('think tank') institution. At a scientific and public education level, the foundation is engaged in the introduction of the paradigm shift on water metabolism of the body in the USA. In his letter (overleaf) Mr Peck briefly explains his medical problems since childhood. Who in the world would have thought so many disparate medical conditions could be related, and after so many years these conditions would disappear as a result of a simple adjustment to daily water intake? The solution to Mr Peck's medical problems was so unique his wife also began to adopt the 'treatment ritual'.

Michael Paturis, the writer of the third letter (see page 77), is a fellow

Rotarian. He became aware of my work when I was asked to speak to his club a few years ago. One day we had lunch and I explained in detail why hypertension and fat accumulation in the body are generally the consequences of chronically occurring dehydration. He accepted my advice of increasing his daily water intake. He also convinced his wife to adopt the measure. Please note the impact of increased water intake on allergies and asthma that has been stated in the letters from Michael Peck and E Michael Paturis.

Lt Col Walter Burmeister has observed the effect of water on his own blood pressure. As you can read in his letter (overleaf), he too

MICRO INVESTMENTS, INC.

Dr. F. Batmanghelidj   25 March 1992
Foundation For The Simple In Medicine
2146 Kings Garden Way
Falls Church, Va. 22043

Dear Fereydoon,
     This letter is a testimony to the merits of water as an essential part of the daily dietary requirements for good health. I have been following your recommendations for nearly five years, and have found myself taking for granted the positive effects of water intake.
     When I first started on the program I was overweight, with high blood pressure and suffering from asthma and allergies, which I have had since a small child. I had been receiving treatment for these conditions. Today, I have my weight and blood pressure under control (weight loss of approximately 30 pounds and a 10 point drop in blood pressure). The program reduced the frequency of asthma and allergy related problems, to the point of practical nonexistence. Additionally, there were other benefits, I experienced fewer colds and flus, and generally with less severity.
     I introduced this program to my wife, who had been on blood pressure medication for the past four years, and through increased water intake has recently been able to eliminate her medication.

     Thanks again for your program,

Michael Peck

has experienced a drug-free and nature-designed adjustment to his blood pressure.

If water is a natural diuretic, why do intelligent and apparently learned people still insist on using chemicals to get rid of water from the kidneys? As far as I am concerned, this constitutes negligence. Since this unfortunate action will eventually damage the kidneys, and ultimately the heart, its practice should stop – to the undoubted benefit of sufferers.

My colleagues who still insist on blindly using diuretics in the treatment of hypertension are walking into foreseeable litigations for

LAW OFFICES OF

E. MICHAEL PATURIS

E. MICHAEL PATURIS

February 20, 1992

LEE STREET SQUARE
431 N. LEE STREET
OLD TOWN
ALEXANDRIA, VIRGINIA 22314

F. Batmanghelidj, M.D.
Foundation For The Simple
  In Medicine
2146 Kings Garden Way
Falls Church, Virginia 22043

Dear Dr. Batmanghelidj:

I again wish to thank you for your kindness in helping my wife and me to better appreciate the importance of water to our health.

We feel the conscious increase in our water consumption contributed greatly to our weight loss -- a weight loss which had been urged upon both of us by our respective physicians for years. My loss of approximately forty-five (45) pounds has resulted in such a lowering of my blood pressure that I am no longer taking medicine for my blood pressure. My wife's weight loss has alleviated the discomfort she has experienced for years with her back. In addition, she believes the weight loss has reduced her discomfort and problems with her allergies.

With best wishes, I remain

Sincerely,

E. Michael Paturis

EMP:map

77

negligent treatment of their patients. The new information will provide their patients with sufficient insight to understand what damage has been caused by stupid insistence on treating 'hypertension' with diuretics. Let the February 1995 class action suit of smokers against the tobacco industry be a warning to the health care industry.

3 August 1994

Dr. Fereydoon Batmanghelidj
Foundation For the Simple in Medicine
2146 Kings Garden Way
Falls Church, Virginia 22043

Dear Dr. Batmanghelidj:

Since my 24 May 1994 letter, and your consequent telephone call, a physical change of address has absorbed my time. The new address is LTC Walter F. Burmeister, 118 Casitas del Este, El Paso, Texas 79935.

Albeit, much more important than these facts, I am in a position to verify how tap water effectively lowers hypertension. Starting in early April 1994, leaving years of diuretics and calcium-blockers behind, in accordance with your recommendation, for approximately 3 months I drank a minimum of eight 8-ounce glasses of tap water; occasionally more. The blood pressure, heretofore contained by drugs, gradually dropped from an average around 150-160 systolic/over 95-98 diastolic to an amazing, drug free, 130-135 systolic/over 75-80 diastolic fluctuating average.

My wife makes these measurements at home; each time taking two or three readings. The record shows several lows of 120s. over 75d. and a rare high of 140s. over 90d. However, the average range, as stated above, uniformly dominates.

In addition to vitamins and minerals, this drug-free approach, based essentially on tap water and a pinch of salt, has relaxed my system and justifies the confidence that you hold the handles of a truly revolutionary and marvelous medical concept.

Since you are about to publish a book with applicable testimonies of the Hydration System, my personal experience is gratefully offered as a way of saying thank you.

Respectfully yours,

Walter F. Burmeister
Lt. Col. AUS RET

118 Casitas del Este Pl.
El Paso, Texas 79935

CHAPTER 7

Higher blood cholesterol

'The secret of caring for a patient
is caring for the patient.'
Sir William Osler

Higher blood cholesterol is a sign that the cells of the body have developed a defence mechanism against the osmotic force of the blood that keeps drawing water out through the cell membranes; or *the concentrated blood cannot release sufficient water to go through the cell membrane* and maintain normal cell functions. Cholesterol is a natural 'clay' that, when poured in the gaps of the cell membrane, will make the cell wall impervious to the passage of water (see Figure 14 overleaf).

Its excessive manufacture and deposition in the cell membrane is part of the natural design for the protection of living cells against dehydration. In living cells that possess a nucleus, cholesterol is the agent that regulates permeability of the cell membrane to water. In living cells that do not possess a nucleus, the composition of fatty acids employed in the manufacture of the cell membrane gives it the power to survive dehydration and drought. Cholesterol production in the cell membrane is a part of the cell survival system. It is a necessary substance. *Its excess denotes dehydration.*

Normally, it is water that instantly, repeatedly and transiently forms into adhesive sheets and binds the hydrocarbon bricks together. In a dehydrated membrane, this property of water is lost. At the same time that water is binding the solid structure of the membrane, it also diffuses through the gaps into the cell.

Figure 14 demonstrates the structure of a bilayer membrane during full hydration and its possible extreme dehydration. I have presented this researched concept at an international gathering of cancer specialists. These same scientific statements are published and have been discussed by other researchers. How does this phenomenon

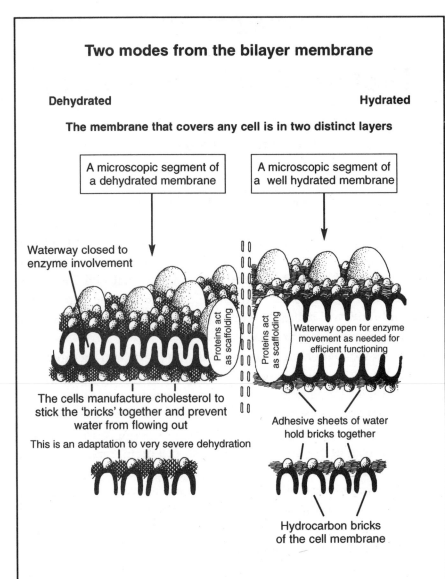

Two modes from the bilayer membrane

Dehydrated   **Hydrated**

The membrane that covers any cell is in two distinct layers

A microscopic segment of a dehydrated membrane

A microscopic segment of a well hydrated membrane

Waterway closed to enzyme involvement

Proteins act as scaffolding

Proteins act as scaffolding

Waterway open for enzyme movement as needed for efficient functioning

The cells manufacture cholesterol to stick the 'bricks' together and prevent water from flowing out

This is an adaptation to very severe dehydration

Adhesive sheets of water hold bricks together

Hydrocarbon bricks of the cell membrane

Figure 14: In a well hydrated membrane, water is the adhesive material that also diffuses through the hydrocarbon 'bricks'. The bilayer is separated and the space is used as a 'waterway' for enzyme activity. In a dehydrated membrane, cholesterol is manufactured to stick the 'bricks' together and also prevents further loss of water from inside the cell. The 'waterway' is also obstructed by the interfit of projections of the bricks – the left side.

affect us in our everyday life? The answer is simple. Imagine that you are sitting at a table and food is brought to you. If you do not drink water before you eat the food, the process of food digestion will take its toll on the cells of the body. Water will have to be poured on the food in the stomach for proteins to break and separate into the basic composition of their amino acids. In the intestine, more water will be required to process the food ingredients and then send them to the liver.

In the liver, the specialised cells will further process the intestine-digested materials and then pass *the resupplied and composition adjusted blood* to the right side of the heart. In the liver, more water is used to process the food ingredients. The blood from the right side of the heart, which has also received some 'fat' components from the lymphatic system that empties into the right side of the heart, will now be pumped into the lungs for oxygenation and exchange of the dissolved gases in the blood. In the lungs, aeration of the blood further dehydrates it by the process of evaporation of water – the 'winter steam'.

Now this highly concentrated blood from the lungs is passed to the left side of the heart and pumped into the arterial circulation. The first cells that will face this highly osmotically concentrated blood are the cells lining the larger blood vessels and capillaries of the heart and the brain. Where the arteries bend, the osmotically damaged cells will also face the pressure of the oncoming blood. Here, the cells will either need to protect themselves or become irreversibly damaged. Do not forget that the integrity of their cell membrane is proportionately dependent on the presence of 'water' available to them and not that which is being osmotically pulled out. A look over the page at Figure 15, then back at Figure 14, should make the process of cholesterol adaptation to dehydration much easier to understand.

There comes a moment when the brain begins to recognise the further imposed severe shortage of water in the body, and then in the middle of eating food the person will feel compelled to drink. It is already too late, because the damage is registered by the cells lining the blood vessels. However, when this dehydration registers itself by

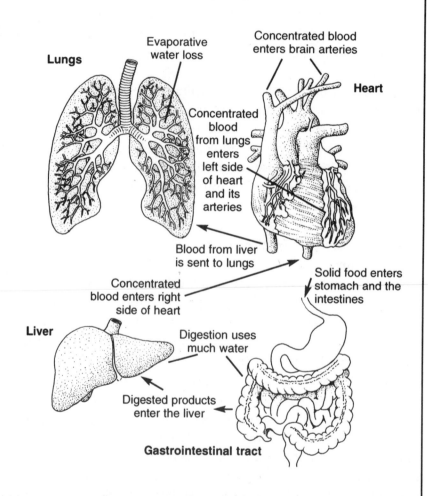

Heart and lungs, the first organs in line of concentrated blood

Figure 15: *Solid foods will be digested in the stomach and the intestines, passed to the liver for further chemical manipulations, and, via the blood circulation through the heart and lungs, will reach the rest of the body. If sufficient water is not taken before food, the circulating blood will be highly concentrated. It will osmotically influence the cells in its path.*

production of the dyspeptic pain, we most stupidly give the person antacid! Not water – antacids! Not water – histamine-blocking agents! Unfortunately, this is the problem with all treatment procedures under the solutes paradigm.

All treatment procedures are oriented towards the relief of symptoms. They are not geared to the elimination of the root cause of the problem. This is why 'diseases' are not cured. They are only 'treated' during the lifetime of the person.

The root cause of degenerative diseases is not known, because a wrong paradigm is being pursued. If we begin to appreciate that for the process of food digestion, *water is the most essential ingredient*, most of the battle is won. If we give the necessary water to the body before we eat food, all the battle against cholesterol formation in the blood vessels will be won.

After a longer period of regulating daily water intake, so that the cells become fully hydrated, gradually the cholesterol defence system against the free passage of water through the cell wall will be less required; its production will decrease. The hormone-sensitive, fat-burning enzymes of the body have been shown to become active after one hour's walk. They remain active for 12 hours. It also seems that with the lowering of blood cholesterol and walking to induce the 'fat burners' activity, deposited cholesterol will also be broken and passage of blood through the already blocked arteries will become possible, as Mr John Fox's letter at the end of this chapter confirms.

Walking twice a day every 12 hours will maintain the activity of the hormone sensitive fat burning enzyme (hormone sensitive lipase) during day and night and help clear away the excess lipid deposits in the arteries.

Testimonials that make you ponder

As a result of my efforts to make the truly beneficial properties of simple tap water more widely known, I receive very many letters from those who have applied my methods and wish to report the results. I value the information in these latters and always read them with great interest, and it is perhaps hardly surprising that the same themes are repeated time after time.

EMBASSY OF THE ARAB REPUBLIC OF EGYPT
PRESS & INFORMATION BUREAU

May 1st, 1991

Dr. Fereydoon Batmanghelidj
Foundation For The Simple In Medicine
P.O Box 3267, Falls Church, VA 22043

Dear Dr. Batmanghelidj,

This is to say how grateful I am to you for making me a much less worried man. I have suffered from a high cholesterol level since 1982. It was 278 when it was first discovered. I was then in Germany and I was put on such a strict diet that I lost 16 pounds in less than two months and the Cholesterol level went down to only 220. I refused to accept to lower it further through medication especially since in Egypt the doctors still believe that this level is not really dangerous by the prevailing standards in our country.

Since I entertain and attend business lunches more than what would be expected even from a diplomat, because of the additional burden of dealing with the media, my cholesterol was always going up to around 260 and back to 220s, by putting myself on very strict diet from time to time. However, it must be noted that it was only outside my home that the diet came crashing down. Otherwise, I was strict with myself. In fact, even when I ate outside, I was careful to choose dishes, wherever available, which were not particularly rich in fat.

Last year I was shocked to discover that my blood cholesterol level had shot up to 279. I was lucky to have met you then. When you "prescribed" ample water (two full glasses) be taken before meals instead of medication that I was just about to submit myself to then, I was very skeptical. All the more so since you did not overemphasize dieting. In two months, and with very little observance of all the old "rules" which were making my life miserable, my cholesterol went down to 203 for the first time in more than nine years! MY weight too was surprisingly also down by about eight pounds and has since been under control. In fact, I feel so good that I am sure that the next time I will be going for a blood test, my cholesterol level will be found to be even lower. So, goodbye to the "normal" Egyptian standards and welcome to the American new levels of cholesterol without the accompanying sense of deprivation!

Enjoying eating, moderately of course, as I had not been doing for a long time and free from a worry that was always at the back of my mind, I believe I owe you a big THANK YOU.

YOURS SINCERELY

MINISTER MOHAMMED WAHBY
Director, Press and Information Bureau

Mr Mohammed Wahby's concern, expressed in the letter opposite, is not unique to him. Everyone who has raised blood cholesterol levels is worried. It is common knowledge that many diseases are associated with raised cholesterol levels in blood circulation. Different blood cholesterol levels have, in the past, been considered normal – all the time decreasing the accepted threshold until around 200 (milligrams per 100 cubic centimetres of blood) is now considered normal. Even this figure is an arbitrary assessment.

I personally believe the normal range to be around 100 to 150. My own levels started around 89 and never went above 130. Why? Because for years and years, my day started with two to three glasses of water. In any case, a March 28, 1991 *New England Journal of Medicine* report, followed by an editorial, about an 88-year-old man who eats 25 eggs daily and has normal blood cholesterol levels, reveals one fact. The cholesterol we eat seems to have little to do with the high level of cholesterol in some people's blood.

Let us get one thing clear: *excess cholesterol formation is the result of dehydration.* It is the dehydration that causes many different diseases and not the level of cholesterol in the circulating blood. It is therefore more prudent to attend to our daily water intake rather than to what foods we eat. With proper enzyme activity, any food can be digested, including its cholesterol content. Mr Wahby could reduce his cholesterol levels without too much anxiety about his food intake.

He lived quite normally and yet his cholesterol levels came down dramatically from 279 to 203 in just two months without any food limitations. All he had to do was to drink more water before his meals. If he had taken regular daily walks, this level would have been further reduced during the two months. In time, it will be further reduced. His testimonial is printed by his kind permission. He is so happy with the simplicity of the process that he wishes to share his joy with others.

If increased water intake lowers cholesterol levels, only to rise again, make sure your body is not getting short of salt. The importance of this is explained in the section on salt that appears in chapter 12. You should realise that cholesterol is the basic building block for

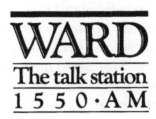

WARD
The talk station
1 5 5 0 · A M

December 2, 1994

Global Health Service, Inc.
Attention: F. Batmanghelidj, M. D.
P. O. Box 3189
Falls Church, VA 22043

Dear Dr. Batmanghelidj:

Just a short letter to thank you for informing our
listeners about the health benefits of drinking two quarts
of water a day.

Not only did you help our radio audience, but I personally
have enjoyed a resurgence of energy after drinking two quarts
of water each day for just over one week.

The angina pain I endured for five years has disappeared and
my distress from a hiatal hernia has greatly lessened. I feel
like a new person.

I've been doing talk shows at WARD Radio for the past 20 years,
and I must say your interview with us is one I'll always
remember.

Sincerely,

WARD Broadcasting Corporation
Samuel M. Liguori, Program Director

SML:rwb

P.O. Box 1550 Pittston, PA 18640

most hormones in the human body. Naturally, a basic drive for increased hormone production will also raise the rate of cholesterol production.

Basically, it is assumed that heart disease begins with the deposit of cholesterol plaques in the arteries of the heart. At the final stages, the two may exist at the same time. However, in my opinion, it begins when the constriction producing chemicals from the lungs spill over into the circulation that goes to the heart.

As we will see in chapter 9, where the subject of asthma is explored, in dehydration, part of the process of water preservation is associated secretion of substances that constrict the bronchioles. At a certain threshold that does not at the time manifest itself in an asthma attack; the same chemicals, if they spill into the blood circulation that goes through to the lung, will also constrict the walls of the heart arteries once they reach them. This situation will lead to heart pains, known as anginal pains.

These same chemicals can also set the stage for the deposit of cholesterol in the walls of the arteries. The common factor to all of the various conditions labelled as different diseases of the heart and the lungs is an established dehydration. Take a look at Mr Sam Liguori's letter (left), published by his kind permission.

His anginal pain disappeared when he started to increase his water intake. He had also suffered from hiatus hernia. That, too, had started to clear up. Given time, and that too might be expected to recover completely.

Then take a look at Loretta Johnson's handwritten letter overleaf. You will see that, even at the age of 90, her anginal pain can be treated with water to the extent that she does not need any medication for her heart pains.

I have many, many letters similar to these. It is simply not possible to publish them all. I have selected a few of them to show you that what I propose is not a theory. It, in fact, works for different people of varying ages.

Mr John Fox's previously quoted case is very unusual in that his severe case of heart disease was reversed sufficiently to make life once again normal for him without the bypass surgery that is now

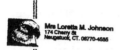

Mrs Loretta M. Johnson
174 Cherry St
Naugatuck, CT. 06770-4585

May 11, 1994

Dear Dr. Batmanghelidj:

I am 90 years old. I have angina. I do not get chest pains or cramps but at the base of my throat I get an ache - a painful tension and my pulse beats like a run-away horse.

But after I read your book "Your Body's Many Cries for Water" I started drinking water. When I get an attack of angina - I rest and drink water! Would you believe it? I don't need the nytro stat (buffered nitroglycerin) anymore. I am so glad because the nitro burned my mouth and gave me oral ulcers. Now I carry a small bottle of water with me at all times in addition to drinking it at home. Thanks a million!

Loretta M. Johnson
Naugatuck, Conn 06770

Mrs Loretta M. Johnson
174 Cherry St
Naugatuck, CT. 06770-4585

so much in vogue. Mr Fox is in his sixth decade of life. He is a retired electronics engineer who has spent many highly responsible years with the Navy.

Today, he is one of the 50 living Bates-Trained Natural Vision specialists. At some point in time, he was nearly blind in one eye and losing vision in the other. He became intrigued with the Bates method of vision training because of his own needs. As a result of his training, he is not going blind any more and his eyesight is saved – it is virtually normal now.

A few years back, he was considered hypertensive. He received medication to reduce his blood pressure. He could not take these medications; they made him worse. His problems started when he suffered his heart attacks. His letter (pages 91 and 92) explains what happened to him and how he is better now.

The highlight of this letter is that after two months of taking increased water, and a slight adjustment to his diet, in addition to his daily walks, his coronary arteries must have cleared sufficiently for him to feel normal. He now enjoys normal activity without having to endure any pain, and all of that without the use of any medication or suffering by-pass surgery.

Imagine that a person with such a severe heart problem as Mr Fox could in about two months get back to normal life and not need any invasive treatment, even though chemical treatments failed! The proposed nature-designed approach to the problem scientifically and logically seems to depend on physiological reversal of the disease process. It's an ideal way of offering *cures* for some degenerative disease conditions.

Adding the statements of Mr Wahby to the results presented by Mr Fox, Mr Paturis, Mr Liguori, Mrs Johnson, Col Burmeister and Mr Peck, one begins to recognise the fact that *common tap water has medicinal values hitherto unrecognised.*

Water is a readily available natural medicine for some prevalent and very serious medical conditions that are known to kill many thousands of people every year. Is it heart disease or dehydration that is killing people? In my professional and scientific view, it is *dehydration* that is the biggest killer, more than any other condition you could imagine. The different physiological aspects and 'chemical idiosyncrasies' of each individual's body reaction to the same pattern of dehydration have received different professional labels and have been treated differently - *and ineffectively.*

Dehydration is the common factor. It is the difference in the 'chemical blueprint' in the design of each person's body that initially demonstrates signs of chronic dehydration by producing different outward indicators.

Later in the process, other indicators of the same dehydration problem become apparent. The reason for this difference in the initial pattern may be the selective process of 'shower-head' emergency hydration of some cell types in the body. If you take a second look at the letters by Mr Peck, Mr Paturis, and read the one from Mr William Gray (on pages 140 to 142), you will see that the individuals in question had multiple problems that got better by the regulation of daily water intake.

You are now privy to information on where the mistake lies in the creation of monstrous problems within the health care systems in scientifically advanced countries. *They seem to allow the arrogant treatment of a simple dehydration of the human body by chemical mallets until real diseases are born.*

BATES-FOX
Natural Vision Training
2945 North Lexington Street Arlington Virginia 22207

Telephone 703 536 7482

Attestation: 25 March 1992

It was in the spring of 1991 when I first learned from a member of the Foundation For the Simple In Medicine the value of water as a form of medication. Six months before, I had suffered two heart attacks and had undergone angioplasty surgery. After the operation, I was prescribed heavy dosages of calcium and beta blockers, baby aspirin, nitroglycerine (for pain), and cholesterol-reducing medicine for recovery. The angiogram before the angioplasty had shown one of the arteries of my heart was 97 percent blocked by cholesterol deposits. I was told my heart had been damaged.

After six months of strict attention to my prescribed "recuperation" program, I noticed that my condition was rapidly deteriorating, to the extent that I had difficulty sleeping because of pain in my left arm, back and chest, and also felt these same pains when I took my daily walks. I visualized myself going for bypass surgery at the scheduled time for reevaluation of my condition. By this time, I also suffered from serious side effects caused by the medications, such as: my prostate created retention and blocking problems; I had also developed problems with my vision and memory recall.

I first began my rehabilitation through diet by a regular intake of six to eight 8-ounce glasses of water each day for three days. I was told to drink water a half-hour before eating my daily meals. I cut off my anti-cholesterol pills, aspirin and nitroglycerine pills. Judging by the effect of the water, it seemed I did not need them. I also started taking orange juice and started using salt in my diet again (I had been on a sodium-free diet). After the first three days, I was feeling more comfortable about all of that added water. After three weeks of gradually reducing the calcium and beta-blockers, I noticed some very favorable changes. Whenever I felt pain, I would drink water and get instant relief. My diet remained the same--fruits, vegetables, chicken, fish, orange juice, and carrot juice. To get more tryptophan, I was asked to add cottage cheese and lentil soup to my diet.

Dr. Batmanghelidj requested that I take two one-hour walks (25 min. mile) a day. After the second month, I noticed no more pain--even walking up steep hills. After the fifth month, I changed my walks to 1/2 hour and increased my pace to a 15-minute mile. No constrictions were noticed during my walks and my energy had increased two-fold. Much of my power to recall had been reestablished, and my vision returned to normal.

In October 1991, I had a series of chemical and physical tests, including x-rays, sonogram, echocardiogram and electro-cardiogram, to determine the state of my heart. The tests showed that my heart had restored to its normal state and I did not need any form of medication to cope with my daily routine. My doctor could not believe how simply all this change had taken place.

John O. Fox

John O. Fox
Bates-Fox Natural Vision Training

CHAPTER 8

Excess body weight

*Q: Why are 30 per cent of Americans overweight?
A: Because of a most basic confusion! They
don't know when they are thirsty; nor do
they know the difference between
'fluids' and 'water'.*

Let us discuss further the letters from Mr Peck and Mr Paturis, as well
as those from Priscilla Preston and Donna Gutkowski that follow in
this chapter. All of them stated they lost between 30 and 45 pounds
in weight when they switched to water as their preferred beverage.
There is another person who gradually lost 58 pounds in less than a
year, weight she had gained in six years. As you read on, you will see
how simply we gain weight. You would think it simplistic if you did
not have the proof in front of you.

The central control system in the brain recognises the low energy
levels available for its functions. The sensations of thirst or hunger
also stem from low, ready-to-access energy levels. To mobilise energy
from that which is stored in the fat, the body needs hormonal release
mechanisms. This process takes a while longer (and some physical
activity for energy release) than the urgent needs of the brain. The
front of the brain either gets energy from 'hydroelectricity' or from
sugar in blood circulation. Its functional needs for hydroelectricity
are more urgent – not only the energy formation from water, but also
its transport system within the microstream flow system that
depends on more water.

Thus, sensations of thirst and hunger are generated simultaneously
to indicate the brain's needs. We do not recognise the sensations of
thirst and assume both to be indicators of the urge to eat. We eat
food even when the body should receive water. In these people who
lost weight, by drinking water before eating food, they managed to

separate the two sensations. They did not overeat to satisfy an urge for the intake of water.

Overeating further explained

The human brain is roughly 2 per cent of the total body weight. It is said to possess about nine trillion nerve cells ('computer chips'). Brain cells are said to be 85 per cent water. Twenty per cent of blood circulation is allocated and made available to the brain. This means that the brain gets to pick and choose from the circulating blood what is needed for its normal functions. The brain is the only part of the body that is constantly active. It processes all information from different parts of the body, as well as that which enters it from daily exposure to physical, social, and *electromagnetic environment.*

To process all these inputs and alert all parts of the body for co-ordinated response, the brain spends a vast quantity of energy. At the same time, it spends energy in manufacturing primary ingredients and different brain chemical messengers (neurotransmitters) that are made in the brain cells and have to be transported to the nerve endings wherever they are. The transport system uses a vast quantity of energy. This high rate of energy consumption by the brain is the main reason for the high level of blood circulation.

Brain cells stockpile energy in two main forms: ATP and GTP reserves like the coal and coke dumps next to power plants. Certain actions are supplied with energy from ATP stockpiles that are located in different parts of the cell, mainly within its membranes. The cell membrane is where the information enters and where an action is initiated. There is a system of energy rationing in operation in each cell. Not all stimulation will achieve an allocation of energy from the ATP stockpile to get registered and invoke a response.

There is a threshold for energy release for some inputs. The brain calculates and understands what is important and what is not for its energy expenditure. When ATP reserves are low, many stimuli do not invoke a response. This low ATP reserve in some overactive brain cells will become reflected as a fatigue state in functions controlled by those brain cells. Exactly the same process is in operation for the GTP stockpiles. In certain emergency actions, some energy from

GTP stockpile can be diverted to boost the ATP stockpile to sustain some of the most essential functions that would otherwise suffer from lack of local energy.

Storage of energy in the brain's energy pools seems to rely heavily on the availability of sugar. The brain is constantly drawing from the blood sugar to replenish its ATP and GTP stockpiles. Recently it has been discovered that the human body has the ability to generate hydroelectric energy when water, by itself, goes through the cell membrane and turns some very special energy generating pumps: very much like the hydroelectric power generation when a dam is built on a large river. Thus, the brain uses two mechanisms for its energy requirements: one, from metabolism of food and formation of sugar; two, from its water supply and conversion of hydroelectric energy. It now seems that the brain depends very extensively on energy formation from hydroelectricity, particularly for its transport system in its nerve supply to different parts of the human body.

To satisfy the brain's requirements, the body has developed a delicate balancing system to keep a normal range of sugar concentration in the blood. It does this in two ways: by stimulating intake of proteins and starchy foods that it will convert to sugar, in addition to the sugar in the diet; by converting some starch and proteins from stored reserves of the body into sugar. This latter mechanism is called gluco-neo-genesis. It means remaking of sugar from other materials. This re-manufacturing of sugar for use by the brain is done in the liver.

The dependence of most brain functions on energy from sugar has developed a satiety or pleasure association with the sweet taste. It has established a certain coding system for co-ordination of functions by the other organs, particularly by the liver when a sweet taste stimulates the tongue. When there is not enough sugar in circulation, the liver begins to manufacture it and constantly tops up blood levels by the addition of more sugar. At the beginning, it will convert stored starch, followed by proteins and small quantities of fat. Fat conversion is a very slow process.

The body needs to go without food for some time before a higher rate of fat metabolism is established. Proteins are more accessible and broken down more easily than fat. Fat deposits are made up of many single units of fatty acids joined together. It is the individual fatty acids that are broken for their energy value. Each gram of fat gives nine calories of energy. Each gram of protein or sugar provides only four calories of energy. This is the reason, when fat is metabolised, that a person is far less hungry.

In children, fat stores are brown in colour and have much blood circulation in them. In brown fat, fat is metabolised directly and heat is generated. In later years of life, fat stores have less blood circulation and are less accessible to the enzymes that would mobilise the fatty acids for conversion in the liver and the muscles. When muscles are inactive, they are more easily attacked and their protein is broken down for conversion into sugar. However, if muscles are used, they begin to metabolise some of their stored fat as a choice source of energy to do work and maintain or increase their bulk. To do this, they begin to activate a fat-breaking enzyme called hormone sensitive lipase. It has been shown in repeated blood tests in Sweden that this enzyme's activity is seen after one hour's walk and retains its fat-breaking activity for 12 hours. Once muscles begin to use fat, more sugar will become available to be used by the brain.

With repeated walks, activity of the fat-burning enzymes become much more pronounced. Thus, a vital component of any dieting programme should be muscle use for its long-lasting, primary and direct physiological effect on fat breakdown. It is this enzyme in blood circulation that will also clean all blood vessel walls of fatty plaques and deposits. It was this physiological response of the body to walking that reversed the health problems of Mr John Fox. Increased water intake gave him energy and stamina and walking stimulated the enzymes that cleared his arteries.

Office work and desk jobs in our modern way of life are only a cultural transformation. The body physiology has not yet transformed sufficiently to accommodate this functionally abnormal use of the human body. The human body still needs muscle activity to maintain normal functions. If the body functions normally, it will know when to eat and how much to eat without storing any fat. Every part of the body will use its share of energy supply for efficient and well-co-ordinated functioning. This is what it is designed for.

However, if the brain is used more (in times of stress) and the body is not used proportionately to supply the brain with its sugar needs, a less-disciplined person will give in to eating more often and in larger quantities. It becomes more dramatic if one does not recognise the other thirst signals of the human body when it needs water for its energy supply, when, in place of drinking water by itself, more food is consumed. In stress, the body becomes dehydrated. The reason we tend to gain weight is one simple fact: we eat to supply the brain with energy for its constant round-the-clock activity. However, when food is eaten, only about 20 per cent of it reaches the brain. The rest will gradually become stored if muscle activity does not use up its allocated portion. With water as a source of energy, this storage does not happen. Excess water is passed out in the form of urine.

Diet sodas can cause weight gain

My observation has been that diet sodas (in this context I am using the term soda for all variety of manufactured soft drinks), even though containing no appreciable number of calories, are possibly the cause of more weight gain in people who resort to taking them to control their weight. One person stands out: a young man in his twenties, about 5ft 5in (1.65m) in height. Like most college students, he used to drink regular sodas while under pressure to complete his studies. He had already gained excess weight by graduation. After graduation, to reduce weight, he upped consumption to eight cans of diet soda per day. In about two years, he must have gained another 30 pounds. He seemed to get as round as he was tall. Walking became difficult, and he seemed to have to swing his hip to take a step. He also drank diet soda at mealtimes and ate more than his body needed. Today, he still consumes his diet sodas – he seems to be addicted – and, despite all other efforts, he continues to be overweight.

This paradox in our understanding of the relationship between taking a sweetener that does not directly contribute to the total calorie intake of the body and weight gain needs explanation. The following is the result of my research into this enigma. There are many people who resort to taking diet sodas and, instead of losing weight, begin to gain it. On page 104, you can read the testimonial from one of them,

Donna Gutkowski, who for years only consumed sodas and gained weight regardless of anything else she did to shed excess pounds.

In America in 1850, about 13 ounces of soda were consumed per person per year. In the late 1980s, more than 500 12-ounce cans of soda were consumed per person per year. The 1994 annual report of the beverage industry shows that per capita consumption of sodas is 49.1 gallons per year. Of this amount, 28.2 per cent of consumption is the share of different diet sodas. Diet soda consumption is beginning to decline. Eighty-four per cent of all sodas consumed belong to two companies (Coca-Cola, 48.2 per cent, and Pepsi-Cola, 35.9 per cent). Of this 84 per cent share of market and the different labels they manufacture, only 5.5 per cent are caffeine-free diet sodas. These figures indicate that a vast number of people are drinking caffeinated sodas, 22 per cent of them diet sodas.

A survey at Pennsylvania State University showed that some students drank 14 cans of soda a day. One girl had consumed 37 Cokes in two days. Many admitted they could not live without soft drinks. If deprived, they would develop withdrawal symptoms, much like those addicted to other drugs. *Boys Life* magazine surveyed readers and found that 8 per cent of them drank eight or more sodas a day. Administrators of one Boy Scout Jamboree collected 200,000 empty cans for recycling. The Soft Drink Association surveyed American hospitals' use of soft drinks and found 85 per cent of them serve sodas with their patients' meals. Research has shown that caffeine is addictive. The media, to placate a beverage industry that spends vast sums of money on advertising its products, have come up with a less expressive word to announce the news. They call it caffeine dependency.

When consumption of sodas is encouraged by society, it is assumed these manufactured beverages can replace the needs of the body for water. It is assumed, just because these beverages contain water, the body will be adequately served. This assumption is wrong. This broad-base increase in consumption of mainly caffeine-containing sodas forms the background to many of the health problems of our society. The mistaken assumption that all fluids are equivalent to water for the water needs of the human body is the main cause of many of the ills of the human body, and it is frequently associated with the initial excessive gain in weight. To understand the above statement, we need to recognise some simple principles of anatomy and physiology of the brain that regulate eating and drinking.

The misapprehension that all manufactured beverages will supply the body with its daily water needs, more than any other cause, is responsible for some of the diseases we encounter. Gross disfigurement of the body by fat collection is the initial step in the decline of the human body, and in my opinion is caused by the wrong choice of fluids intake. Some of these beverages do more damage than others.

Caffeine, one of the main components of most sodas, is a drug. It has addictive properties because of its direct action on the brain. It also acts on the kidneys and causes increased urine production. Caffeine has diuretic properties. It is, physiologically, a dehydrating agent. This characteristic is the main reason a person is forced to drink so many cans of soda every day and never be satisfied. The water does not stay in the body long enough. At the same time, many people confuse their feeling of thirst for water: thinking they have consumed enough 'water' that is in the soda, they assume they are hungry and begin to eat more than their body's need for food. Thus, dehydration caused by caffeine-containing sodas will, in due time, cause a gradual gain in weight from overeating as a direct result of confusion of thirst and hunger sensations.

Caffeine has 'pick-me-up' properties. It stimulates the brain/body even when a person is exhausted! It seems that caffeine lowers the threshold of ATP stockpile control. Stored ATP is used up for some functions that would not normally gain access to it when there is a set level of reserves. When sodas contain sugar, at least some of the brain's need for sugar is satisfied. If caffeine is releasing ATP energy to enhance performance, at least its sugar companion will replenish some of the lost ATP, even if the final result is a deficit expenditure of ATP by the brain.

In the early 1980s, a new product called aspartame was introduced into the beverage industry, as an artificial sweetener other than saccharin. Aspartame is 180 times sweeter than sugar without any calorie output and it is now in common use because the Food and Drug Administration (FDA) has deemed it safe to use in place of sugar. In a very short period of time, it has been incorporated in over five thousand recipes.

In the intestinal tract, aspartame converts to two highly excitatory neurotransmitter amino acids: *aspartate* and *phenylalanine*, as well as methyl alcohol/formaldehyde wood alcohol. It is claimed the liver renders methyl alcohol non-toxic. I personally think this claim is made to brush aside voiced objections for commercialisation of a manufactured 'food' that has a *known toxic by-product*.

If caffeine converts ATP to AMP, a spent energy 'ash', aspartate converts GTP energy stockpile to GMP. Both AMP and GMP are spent fuels; they cause thirst/hunger to replace the lost fuel stockpiles in the brain cells. Thus, diet sodas cause indiscriminate overuse of the energy reserves of cells in the brain.

It is a well recognised, scientific fact that spent fuel AMP causes hunger. Caffeine causes addiction, and people who consume it on a regular basis should be assumed to be 'sodaholics'. Hence, caffeinated diet sodas used by sedentary persons must cause weight gain; they indirectly stimulate more food intake because of the brain's forced use of its energy reserves. Bear in mind that only some of the energy value of foods eaten will be used by the brain. The rest of the consumed energy will be stored as fat if it is not used by muscle activity. This weight gain is one of many results of diet soda consumption.

The more important reflex that occurs is a brain reaction to sweet taste. The term used to describe this is *cephalic phase response*. A conditioned reflex becomes well established as a result of lifelong experience with sweet taste that is associated with the introduction of new energy into the body. When sweet taste stimulates the tongue, the brain programmes the liver to prepare for acceptance of new energy – sugar – from outside. The liver, in turn, stops the manufacture of sugar from the protein and starch reserves of the body and instead begins to store the metabolic fuels that are circulating in the blood. As Michael G Tardoff, Mark I Friedman, and other scientists have shown, cephalic phase responses alter the metabolic activity in favour of nutrient storage; the fuel available for conversion is reduced which leads to the development of appetite.

If it is indeed sugar that stimulates the response, the effect on the liver will be the regulation of that which has entered the body. But if sweet taste is not followed by nutrient availability, an urge to eat will be the outcome. It is the liver that produces the signals and the urge to eat. The more sweet taste without accompanying calories that stimulates the taste buds, the more urge there is to eat – or overeat.

The effect of cephalic phase response to sweet taste has been clearly shown in animal models with the use of saccharin. Using aspartame, several scientists have shown a similar urge to overeat in humans. Blundel and Hill have shown that non-nutritive sweeteners – aspartame – in solution will enhance appetite and increase short-term food intake. They report: 'After ingestion of aspartame, the volunteers were left with a residual hunger compared with what they reported after glucose. This residual hunger is functional, it leads to increased food consumption.'

Tardoff and Friedman have shown that this urge to eat more food after artificial sweeteners can last up to 90 minutes after the sweet drink; even when all blood tests show normal values. They showed that even when blood levels for insulin – the higher readings of which is thought to be the cause of hunger – achieved normal levels, test animals consumed more food than the control batch. What this means is that, for a long time, the brain retains the urge to eat when the taste buds for sugar are stimulated without sugar having entered the system. The sweet taste will cause the brain to programme the liver to store supplies rather than release supplies from its storage.

Basically, this physiological response to sweeteners without the accompanying calories that the body believes have entered will compel the person to find and make good the registered marker for energy consumption. This is another physiological reason why people who consume diet sodas to reduce weight may suffer from the paradoxical response of their body to repeated stimulation of the taste buds with sugar substitutes.

When caffeine and aspartame are introduced into the body, they will stimulate the cell physiology in the brain, the liver, the kidneys, the pancreas, the endocrine glands, and so on. Aspartame is converted to phenylalanine and aspartate. Both have direct stimulatory effects on the brain. The sum total of the effect of caffeine and aspartame will very quickly establish a new mode of activity for the brain just because they are repeatedly available in larger quantities than the ones that would otherwise establish a balanced physiology.

Most neurotransmitters are secondary products from one or another amino acid. However, aspartate is one of a pair of unique amino acids that don't need to be converted to a secondary product to cause an effect on the brain. There are receiving points (receptors) for these two stimulant amino acids (aspartate and glutamate) on certain nerve cells that influence body physiology very dramatically.

The use of artificial sweeteners for their false stimulation of 'nerve terminals' that register the entry of energy supplies into the body have more severe repercussions than simply causing an increase in weight. These chemicals constantly swing the body physiology in the direction dictated by the nerve system they stimulate. Their use without a thorough understanding of their long-term effects in the body, just because they also pleasantly stimulate the taste buds, is short-sighted. My understanding of the microphysiology within cells causes me concern when I think of the routine use of these amino acids. I worry about the long-term effect of direct stimulation of the nerve/glandular systems in the brain with these chemical sweeteners. These systems are naturally positioned for other important, but balanced functions, in the body.

Research has shown that receptors for aspartate are abundantly present on some nerve systems whose products also stimulate the reproductive organs and breasts. Constant stimulation of breast glands without the other factors associated with pregnancy may well be implicated in the rising rate of breast cancer in women. The hormone, prolactin, may play a major role in this. One of the less explored complications of aspartame may be its effect as a possible facilitator in cancer formation in the brain. Fed to rats, aspartame has been implicated in the formation of brain tumours in experimental animals.

As an analogy, imagine a small sail boat that is going from one port to another nearby and has to reach its destination before dark, when the direction of the winds is not ideal. If the sailor, instead of paying strict attention to the rules of sailing, gives in to the pleasure and exhilaration of fast sailing with the wind, he will have abandoned his purpose and sailed his boat to totally different and unknown shores, and end up in the dark. The odds are that he and his boat will not survive the trip. On its journey of life, the human body is like that sail boat. If the mind abandons its purpose and forgets the design of the body, and gives in to the overstimulation of the palate with artificial and non-representative products (such as spices), *in the long run,* the body chemistry may not be able to deal with constant false information without suffering damage.

It is primitive and simplistic thinking that one could easily lace water with all sorts of pleasure-enhancing chemicals and substitute these fluids for the natural and clean water that the human body needs. Some of these chemicals – caffeine, aspartame, saccharin and alcohol – through their constant lopsided effect on the brain, unidirectionally, or single-mindedly, programme body chemistry with results contrary to the natural design of the body. Very much like the sail boat in the dark that will get beached in uncharted shores, the intake of wrong fluids will affect the life of anyone who continually consumes them.

As has been explained so far, the human body has many different indicators of when it runs short of water. At these times, it needs only water. It only complicates matters if one gives the body artificial taste-enhancing fluids on a regular basis and in full substitution of the water needs of the body.

One should remember that caffeine, similarly, is an addictive drug, albeit a legal one. Children, in particular, become vulnerable to the addictive properties of caffeine-containing beverages. Stimulating the body in the early stages of life with pleasure-enhancing chemicals in beverages will, in some children, programme the senses to use harder addictive drugs when they reach school age.

The long-term and constant use of sodas in general, and diet sodas in particular, should be assumed to be responsible for some of the more serious health problems of our society. Distorting the physical appearance of the body as a result of excess fat storage is the first step in this direction. Some manufactured beverages should only be used sparingly by young people, if at all, when the right programme for the future health of a child is the aim of parents.

Dr Marcia Gutkowski is a nutrition consultant. After reading my book, she convinced her daughter Donna to begin changing her fluid intake habits. The result astounded both mother and daughter. The following is the transcript of Donna's testimonial.

April 25, 1994
Dear Dr Batmanghelidj
My mother asked that I write to you and tell you about my recent weight loss success. I know that I could have a much more successful loss if I would follow your formula and curb my eating habits, along with starting a regular routine of exercise. However just getting myself to get off of six to eight cans of Mountain Dew a day is a miracle in itself.

Within the last nine months to a year, I have successfully been able to keep 35 excess pounds of baggage off. I am able to wear clothes that I thought would never touch my body again. I also have just about reached my goal size for my upcoming wedding. Even my fiancé had to admit that I am looking much better than when he first met me five years ago.

My success has been contributed to faithfully drinking half my body weight in ounces in water every day. Wherever I go, so does my water. To work, shopping, even my long seven hour long car rides. (That does make for a lot of rest area stops, but they are worth it.) I do treat myself to an occasional mineral water or beer when I go out, but I have usually gotten my quota of water in for the day.

One interesting thing that I have noticed, however, is that once I have finished drinking my quota of water, I have absolutely no desire to drink anymore. Also I have found that I'm not thirsty anymore and it will usually take me awhile to drink some other type of beverage whether it be juice, milk, beer, mineral water, etc.

I am looking forward to October 1st which is my wedding day when I can walk down the aisle looking better than I have looked in 15 years, since I graduated from high school. It will also be nice to put my weight on my new driver's license without having to cringe for the first time in my life.

Thanks for the smaller me!!!!
Donna M Gutkowski

Donna is now happily married; by the time of her wedding in October 1994, she had lost over 40 pounds.

This science-based way of weight loss will be permanent, whereas with a programme of food limitation only, even if some weight is lost, it is regained in a short period of time. Worse still, people are constantly hounded by the fallacy of needing to limit this or that type of food, particularly the cholesterol content of food, which is a temporary present-day vogue.

Do not be shocked – but contrary to the present trend for the exclusion of eggs from a 'healthy' daily diet, I actually eat as many eggs as I feel like eating with no limitation whatsoever. Eggs have a very well balanced protein content, and I also happen to understand how excess cholesterol formation in the body is associated with prolonged dehydration.

Priscilla Preston's following letter (overleaf) further explains the relationship of dehydration, not only to weight gain, but to the more devastating problem of asthma, the subject of the next chapter. In taking steps to prevent asthma, she also managed to lose 35 pounds. Another important point in her letter is the role of salt in disease prevention. Salt is important to the body. Salt sensors on the tongue, when strongly stimulated, remove the body's anxiety and stop it from panicking for water. When salt is available, the body is at least assured of an efficient water filtration system for its emergency supply to the important cells. You will read more about the importance of salt in chapter 12.

Please bear in mind that these letters are real-life stories. They are not anecdotes. We do not need statistics to convince people of the efficacy of water, when the body is clearly demonstrating an urgent need for it. *Whose fault is it that the human body's regional calls for water, and its programme of adaptation to dehydration, have been labelled as disease conditions?* Is there any plausible reason why, for evaluation of natural treatment procedures, we should adhere to the self-serving methodology and the yardstick of the pharmaceutical industry? Their inaccurate assertions have until now caused so much pain and agony for people whose bodies were only crying out for water!

October 31, 1994

To Whom It May Concern:

Priscilla D. Preston, APR

Public Relations

1232 South Crockett

Amarillo, Texas 79102

(806) 374-3123

Imagine having to sleep in an upright position for almost a year, struggling for each breath and suffering from countless asthma and panic attacks nightly! That was me until five months ago! On March 27, 1993 I was hospitalized with a severe asthma attack and developed bronchial pneumonia! My blood gases registered 40 and I was in a life-threatening situation!

After my release from the hospital, I was placed on large doses of theophyllin and prednisone. My **weight skyrocketed** and the medication caused me to become hostile and disoriented. I really didn't want to live! Then, a wonderful friend gave me a flyer on Dr. Batmanghelidj's book *Your Body's Many Cries for Water!* I quickly mailed a check and a letter to the doctor, pleading for a fast delivery! To my complete surprise, he called me personally and started helping me by telephone to get off the medication, which was inappropriate for my condition at this time and asked me to drink at least three liters of water a day and use a small amount of salt! He also asked me to walk in an indoor shopping mall for 15 minutes a day. I can now walk for 30 minutes a day and my breathing is 100% better!

As of this date, October 31, 1994, I am no longer on any medicaton for asthma! I have not used an inhaler or medication of any sort for more than five months! When I start any sort of mild wheezing, I just drink a glass of water and take a little salt and I'm fine!

And....guess what? All of the wonderful water and walking has made me lose 35 lbs. I'm now back to my desired weight and I look young, vibrant and healthy again!

There are millions of Americans out there who need to get "the message." They suffer from AIDS, asthma, arthritis and chronic fatigue syndrome, etc. Everyone in America could benefit from reading Dr. Batmanghelidj's books!

Very sincerely,

Priscilla Preston

CHAPTER 9

Asthma and allergies

It is estimated that 12 million American children suffer from asthma, and several thousand die every year. Let us declare an end to asthma in less than five years. Let us save children from the constant fear of suffocation because they do not recognise they are thirsty for water!

Asthma and allergies are indicators that the body has resorted to an increase in production of the neurotransmitter histamine, the sensor regulator of water metabolism and its distribution in the body. It is recognised that asthmatics have an increase in histamine content of their lung tissue and that it is the histamine that regulates the bronchial muscle contraction. Since one of the sites for water loss through evaporation is in the lungs, bronchial constriction produced by histamine means less water evaporation during the act of breathing – a simple natural manoeuvre to preserve the body's water.

Histamine is an agent that, apart from its water regulatory role, has responsibilities in antibacterial, antiviral, and anti-foreign agents (chemicals and proteins) defence systems in the body. At a normal level of water content of the body, these actions are at an imperceptive or unexaggerated level. At a dehydrated state of the body, to the point where histamine activity becomes exaggerated for water regulation, an immune system activation of histamine-producing cells will release an exaggerated amount of the transmitter that is held in storage for its other functions.

It has been shown in animal models that histamine production in histamine-generating cells will decrease with an increase in the daily water intake. Both of these conditions should be regulated with an alert and determined increase in water intake. On average, these

VON KIEL FAMILY MEDICINE & WELLNESS CENTER

Erik Von Kiel, D.O.   *Board Certified Family Practice with emphasis on Preventive Medicine*

Liberty Square Medical Center
501 North 17th Street • Suite 200
Allentown, PA 18104
(610) 776-7639

1/6/95

Jose A. Rivera M.D.
Lecturer/Member Advisory Board
International Federation of Holistic Medicine

Dr. F. Batmanghelidj
Global Health Solutions
Falls Church, VA. 22043

Dear Dr. Batmanghelidj
    This letter is in appreciatiion for the information that you have presented concerning water dehydration and asthma. As you recall I have had adult onset asthma since I was in college and have had many bouts of anaphylaxis which were life threatening.
    Due to the information that you have provided I have been able to ameliorate and cure my own asthma with water and salt intake. I have been asthma free for approximately 1.5 years and have not had any reactions to the allergens of the past.
    The information has been most helpful in making me aware of when and how to drink water and take salt inorder to hydrate myself and prevent any recurrence of asthma.
    Also, I have been able to advise other patients with respiratory and allergen problems in how to increase their water and salt intake safely, and to my amazement the amelioration has been dramatic.
    Thank you sir for giving me and others the breath of life thru something so simple as water and salt.
    Sincerely,

Jose A. Rivera M.D.

conditions respond after one to four weeks of water regulation of the body.

Mr Michael Peck, who is quoted in Chapter 6, describes being an asthmatic since childhood. He also became sensitive to all sorts of 'allergens', but is no longer in fear of these health problems. Also in Chapter 6, Mr Michael Paturis testified to the fact that his wife's allergic condition became less problematic.

Jose Rivera, MD (see letter opposite), had for years suffered from allergies and asthma. He was severely allergic to cats. In fact, he would never go to a house where a cat was kept. It seems he at one time got very sick after being exposed to a cat. As a result of using the new information about the relationship of dehydration to excess histamine production in the body, he has totally recovered from both of these conditions. To top it all, he now treats asthmatics with water and salt.

Priscilla Preston's letter you have already seen (page 106). Joanie Winfield's letter is printed overleaf. I only discuss these people because their letters testify to the fact that increased daily water intake has provided total relief from asthma and allergies in adults, even after many years of suffering from the problem.

Do not forget that, if concentrated blood reaches the lungs, *local histamine production is a natural and automatic process.* Its exaggerated release will promote bronchial constriction. If you suffer from asthma or allergies, increase your daily water intake. *Do not overdrink, thinking you can undo the damage of many months or years of dehydration by excessive intake of water in a few days. You need to drink a normal amount every day - eight to ten eight-ounce glasses - until full hydration of the body is achieved over a longer period of time.*

Reduce orange juice intake to one or, at most, two glasses a day, because the potassium content of orange juice is high. High loads of potassium in the body can promote higher than average histamine production. In asthmatics, this point should be kept in mind.

Mary B is one of the administrators in a government department that is responsible for the health care system of a major city. She suffered from asthma for many years. She no longer enjoyed her

Joanie Winfield
206 West Prospect Avenue
Pittsburgh, PA 15205
(412) 922-1625

July 18, 1994

Fereydoon Batmanghelidj, M.D.
2146 Kings Garden Way
Falls Church VA 22043

Dear Dr. Batmanghelidj:

I am writing this letter to thank you for sharing your
discovery about the need for water with your readers. I
have benefited greatly from following your advice on water
intake.

The changes in my health have been very noticable. Asthma
used to be a major health concern of mine. Since I have
been drinking enough water, however, I have been able to
breath fine without the use of any medicine. What a difference
this has made in my life. There have been other benefits
as well, such as softer skin and increased mental awareness.

I am so happy to have read your book, and I share your advice
with as many people as I can. Once again, thank you for
your help.

Sincerely,

Joanie Winfield

Joanie Winfield

walks in the parks. Shortness of breath deprived her of the joys of walking. It just so happened that one of my colleagues at the Foundation for the Simple in Medicine became aware of her problem. Responding to the recommendation to drink water, she indicated she was taking ample water. When she was asked to define her daily water intake, it came to light that she was drinking many glasses of *orange juice* and was counting her juice intake as *water* intake. It was explained to her that, although orange juice contains *water*, it cannot be assumed it *replaces* the needs of the body for pure and simple water. She accepted the advice to cut the juice intake and increase her water intake. Within days her shortness of breath improved. The last time we heard from her, she was apparently clear of her asthma.

Let me explain another very important issue in asthma – that is, the role of salt. When there is a water shortage, the body begins to retain salt. But in some people the salt-regulatory mechanisms are inefficient. To this physiological problem may be added bad education about dieting and salt-free diets that have become established trends in our society. In certain people, salt shortage in the body can occur and become symptom-producing in exactly the same way as water shortage, such as some arthritis pains.

It is my understanding that in severe asthma attacks, salt shortage is a major contributing factor. *I would like to share an important secret with you. Salt is a natural antihistamine. People with allergies should begin to increase their salt intake to prevent excess histamine production.*

Water is needed in the lungs to keep the air passages moist and prevent them from drying up when air goes in and comes out. In dehydration, mucus secretion protects air passages from drying. In the first stages of asthma, mucus is secreted to protect the tissues. There comes a time when much mucus is secreted and it stays put, preventing normal passage of air through the airways. Sodium is a natural mucus breaker, and it is normally secreted to make mucus 'disposable'. That is why phlegm tastes salty when it comes in contact with the tongue.

Salt is needed to break up the mucus in the lungs and render it

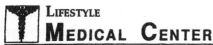

LIFESTYLE
MEDICAL CENTER
Family Medicine • Reconstruction Therapy for Back, Knee, Hand and Joint Pain • Varicose Vein Therapy

Dr. Batmanghelidj   May 24, 1995
2146 Kings Garden Way
Falls Church, VA 22043

                          Reference: Jeremy Christopher
Dear Dr. Batmanghelidj:

I am writing to thank you for your kind assistance in treating Jeremy's allergies. As you know, Jeremy is my eight year-old son who suffered for the last 3-4 years with severe allergy symptoms related to allergic rhinitis and asthma.

More Recently he has had significant coryza and coughing which is associated with his asthma. On about the 28th of April 1995, we began a program of rehydration involving his drinking two cups of water before food or exercise and excluding all other fluids. In addition, he consumes a half teaspoon of salt which is added to his food to offset the increased water intake.

Within 3-4 days he showed dramatic improvement; he no longer had severe and excessive mucus production, his coughing had virtually stopped, and his sneezing and other allergy symptoms were totally gone. Therefore we discontinued his Benadryl and Albuterol and continued his hydration program.

Jeremy has been following this program now for approximately four and a half weeks, spending almost four weeks off his medication and is doing quite well. Not only have his symptoms cleared subjectively, but in terms of objective findings, his peak flow volumes have been within normal range. His constant medication-induced drowsiness has disappeared and as a result he is more alert, and his school grades have improved.

Therefore I want to emphasize how effective this treatment has been for Jeremy and I wish you well in sharing this cost effective and very efficacious program with others.

Once again Dr. Batmanghelidj, I thank you for advising me on the new treatment program of Jeremy's allergies and asthma.

Very truly yours,

Cheryl Brown-Christopher, M.D.

1419 Forest Drive • Suite #202 • Annapolis • Maryland 21403 • (410) 268-5005

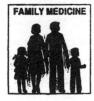
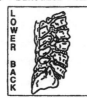
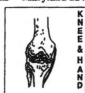
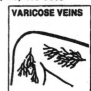

112

watery for its expulsion from the airways. In dehydration, and in conjunction with water preservation mechanisms, a simultaneous and associated salt-preservation programme is established. Not losing salt to mucus secretion becomes part of the programme. The body needs to be assured that both water and salt are available before bronchial constriction relaxes and mucus becomes loose enough to be secreted.

In children with fibrocystic lungs, this relationship of salt and water for normal lung development and functions, as well as mucus secretion, should be kept in mind.

This is why Priscilla Preston's and Dr Rivera's asthma got better. This is why asthma is not a 'disease' that needs to be 'cured'. It is a physiological adaptation of the body to dehydration and salt shortage. It will recur whenever insufficient attention is paid to regular water and salt intake.

A pinch of salt on the tongue after drinking water fools the brain into thinking a lot of salt has arrived in the body. It is then that the brain begins to relax the bronchioles. Alcohol and caffeine contribute to severe asthma attacks. People with asthma should slightly increase their salt intake.

Read Dr Christopher's letter to me (opposite). Her son, Jeremy, was on two different medications for his asthma. The air capacity of his lungs, even with medications, was 60 per cent of normal. In one month of water and salt treatment, his lung capacity went to 120 per cent of normal, with no medication.

Consider also the case of Aaron Warner. At 10 years of age he was put on five different medications intended to treat his asthma. In his mother's words to me: 'The schedule my son would need to keep to maintain his medications was not very realistic for a ten-year-old, and after two days on medications he was feeling worse and his head hurt, throat hurt, mouth hurt and he was tired, drowsy, grouchy and became sun-sensitive.'

As a result of water and salt treatment, Aaron, too, was able to come off medication. The parents of both Jeremy and Aaron are elated, and the information that salt and water can cure asthma was aired for the first time on 5 June 1995 by Paul Harvey News.

This good news is now becoming more and more widely known.We may be able to end in less than five years the scourge of medical ignorance about chronic dehydration that permits so many millions of innocent children to suffer unnecessarily to the point of several thousand a year dying of asthma.What parents need to realise is the fact that breathing becomes difficult for asthmatic children because they are so thirsty.

Multiply the impact on 12 million asthmatic children of increased water intake to prevent asthma attacks and you can suddenly see the possibility of saving them all from 'suffocation and death' from dehydration.

But it can only be done quickly with your active help, and if we can get the media to lend a hand in educating the public about the role of water in the prevention of asthma. Otherwise suffering children will remain in the grip of ignorance and commercialism in medicine.

CHAPTER 10

Some metabolic aspects of stress and dehydration

'I firmly believe that if the entire materia medica *as now used could be sunk to the bottom of the sea, it would be all the better for mankind and all the worse for the fishes.'*
Oliver Wendell Holmes

Insulin-independent diabetes

Basically, there are two types of diabetes. For the treatment of one, insulin is needed because the pancreas no longer manufactures insulin. This type is called *insulin-dependent or Type I diabetes.* For treatment of the other, some chemicals are needed that can gradually release insulin from the pancreas so the diabetic can control the clinical symptoms. This type is called *insulin-independent or Type II diabetes;* the pancreas still has the ability to manufacture insulin.

Insulin-independent diabetes, often established in the elderly and regulated by the intake of tablet forms of medication, is most probably the end result of brain water-deficiency, to the point that its neuro-transmitter systems – particularly the serotonergic system – is being affected. The physiology of the brain is designed in such a way that it automatically begins to peg-up the glucose threshold, so that it can maintain its own volume and its own energy requirements. The brain needs glucose for its energy value and its metabolic conversion to water. The prevalent consensus of opinion is that the bulk of energy requirement in the brain is provided by sugar alone. My personal view is that this is only the case if there is water and salt shortage in the body. Water and salt are absolutely essential for the generation of hydroelectric energy, particularly for neurotransmission mechanisms.

The reason and the mechanism for altering blood sugar levels are quite simple. When histamine becomes active in water regulation and energy management, it also activates a group of substances known as *prostaglandins* (PGs). PGs are involved in a subordinate system for rationed distribution of water to the cells in the body.

The pancreas is a complex gland located between the stomach and the duodenum and, other than being the seat of insulin manufacture, it is engaged in the production of copious quantities of a bicarbonate-containing watery solution. This bicarbonate solution is emptied into the duodenum to neutralise acid coming from the stomach. The acid from the stomach is neutralised while the stimulating agent, PG of the E type, is involved in shunting circulation to the pancreas so the watery bicarbonate solution can be made. At the same time, it naturally inhibits the secretion of insulin from the pancreas. It acts like a very tightly operated servo-mechanism. The more that one system has to be served, the more the other system will be decommissioned.

Why? Quite simply, insulin promotes the movement of potassium and sugar into the cells of the body. It also promotes the entry of some amino acids into cells. Accompanying the passage of sugar, potassium, and amino acids, water also passes into the cell stimulated by insulin. Such action automatically reduces the available water that is more easily accessible from outside the cells. In a dehydrated state, the action of insulin would be counterproductive.

The logic employed in the design of the body has therefore installed the two actions of water distribution to the pancreas and the needed inhibition of insulin action in the same agent prostaglandin E. In this way, and at the expense of severe deprivation of some cells, water is made available for the act of food digestion and acid neutralisation in the intestines.

As it happens, when insulin secretion is inhibited, the metabolism of the body is severely disrupted, with the exception of the brain. In a dehydrated state, the brain benefits from insulin inhibition. The brain cell itself is not dependent on insulin for its functions, while cells in most other parts of the body are totally dependent on the properties of insulin for their normal function. If we think about it, there is a natural logic to the ultimate production of insulin-independent diabetes in severe chronic dehydration. So why is this known as insulin-independent diabetes? Because the body can still manufacture insulin, although it takes the influence of some chemical agents to promote its secretion.

This phenomenon of insulin inhibition with dehydration shows that the primary function of the pancreatic gland is directed at the provision of water for food digestion. Insulin inhibition is an adaptation process of the gland to the dehydration of the body.

Tryptophan and diabetes

Even the simplest explanation of tryptophan may seem complicated! However, basic understanding about this amino acid is needed to make sense of some of the statements presented in this book. Remember, the body is a very complex chemical plant that is extremely sensitive to fluctuations in the flow of its primary raw materials.

The brain is designed to resuscitate itself *when there is water and salt shortage in the body* by raising the levels of sugar in circulation. The raised level of sugar is supposed to balance the vital osmotic equilibrium, in the same way that a doctor resuscitates a patient by the use of sugar and salt-containing intravenous fluid drips. One also needs to recognise another simple point: osmotic forces that must be available for extracellular fluid volume regulation are developed primarily by its salt content, by its raised sugar content, and sometimes by its increased uric acid content.

But in the insulin-dependent type of diabetes there may be severe salt shortage, in which case the brain has no alternative but to raise the level of sugar even more to compensate for the low salt reserves in the body. This process is an automatic step in the design of brain activity master-managed by the various direct, and indirect, functions of tryptophan. It has also been shown that tryptophan is the basic substance the body needs as a vital ingredient to convert into the three or even four most essential neurotransmitters so far recognised.

In insulin-independent diabetes, one must pay particular attention to adequate protein intake to make up for the possible *tryptophan insufficiency* that may be the root cause of the disease. Why? It seems that *dehydration causes severe depletion of brain tryptophan*, an essential amino acid in the human body. When there is an adequate amount of tryptophan in the brain, among its other effects, the pain threshold is raised. *The level of tryptophan content in the brain shows a great drop in some diabetic animals.*

To stress this point again, salt, sugar, and uric acid are involved in balancing the osmotic forces of fluid composition held outside the cells. Salt content is responsible for the greatest contribution to the extracellular osmotic balance. Regulatory properties of tryptophan itself, or its dependent neurotransmission systems, operate a measuring mechanism for the amount of salt that is kept in the body. Serotonin, tryptamine, melatonin, and indolamine are derived from tryptophan, and all are neurotransmitters. Thus, *tryptophan is the natural brain regulator for salt absorption in the body.* It seems that lower levels of tryptophan – and in consequence, its neurotransmitter products – will establish lower-than-normal salt reserves.

As a back-up mechanism in the body, the RA system seems to compensate by inducing salt retention in the body. Histamine and its RA system activity become increasingly engaged if the tryptophan-dependent neurotransmitter systems become less involved through shortage or increased breakdown of tryptophan. It follows that a low-salt diet is not conducive to the correction of a diabetic's high blood sugar.

If the blood sugar is to come down, a slight upward adjustment of daily salt intake may become unavoidable.

Tryptophan is also a prominent amino acid employed in the correction of errors in the process of DNA 'printout' or replica production. With another amino acid, lysine, they form a bridging system (lysine-tryptophan-lysine tripod) that cuts and splices the inaccuracies in DNA transcription. *This property of tryptophan is essential to prevention of cancer cell development in the body.*

With the brain's tryptophan replenishment, the histamine-operated systems will be trimmed down to their primary responsibilities – unexaggerated functions. Salt content of the body will become better regulated. The sensation level before registering pain stimulus will be raised. Acid secretion in the stomach will come under normal control. Blood pressure will be normalised to its natural levels for the operation of all functions in the body: kidneys, brain, liver, lungs, gastrointestinal digestive activities, 'shower-head' filtration of water into the nerve cells, the joints, and so on will function within their normal range of activity.

There is a direct relationship between walking and the build-up of the brain tryptophan reserves. There are several amino acids that compete for crossing the naturally designed barrier system into the brain. They all have to 'piggyback' on the same transporter proteins. These competitors to tryptophan are grouped under the title of branched-chain amino acids (BC amino acids). During exercise, these *BC amino acids,* along with the fats, are used as fuel in the larger muscles. Muscles begin to pick up these amino acids from circulating blood. As a result, the odds are changed in favour of tryptophan for its passage across the blood-brain barrier and into the brain. One major physiological value to exercising is the direct relationship of muscle activity to the build-up of the brain tryptophan reserves.

The brain tryptophan content and its various by-product neurotransmitter systems are responsible for maintenance of the homeostatic balance of the body. Normal levels of tryptophan in the brain maintain a well-regulated balance in all functions of the body: homoeostasis. With a decrease in tryptophan supply to the brain, there is a proportionate decrease in the efficiency of all functions in the body.

Depression and some mental disorders are the consequence of brain tryptophan imbalance. Prozac, which is used in some mental disorders – particularly in depression – is a drug that stops the enzymes that break down serotonin, a by-product of tryptophan. When more serotonin is present, all nerves function normally. But Prozac cannot replace the indispensable role of tryptophan itself. *One has to work at replenishing body reserves of tryptophan through a balanced diet and regular water intake.*

My research has shown there is a direct relationship between water intake – haemodilution – and *efficiency* of function in the transport system for the passage of tryptophan into the brain. Water shortage and proportionate histamine release bring about an increase in the rate of tryptophan breakdown in the liver. It seems that adequate water intake arrests the increased and inefficient metabolism of tryptophan in the body. Chronic dehydration causes its loss from the pool of different amino acids held in the body. Tryptophan cannot be manufactured in the body; it must be imported through food intake. It is one of the essential amino acids. Thus, hydration of the body, *exercise* and the intake of right foods help replenish brain tryptophan reserves.

It is most important to remember the idiosyncrasies that seem to operate in protein metabolism and their manufacture. Proteins are manufactured from joining amino acids together. There are 20 amino acids (AAs) from which different proteins are made. Each protein has a different mix of these AAs. Depending on the sequence of the mix, different characteristics are installed in each protein. Depending on the sequence and the number, the mix can function as enzymes, as assembly lines for the manufacture of other proteins, and as energy generators in the hydroelectric pump units.

All functions of the body are regulated by the special properties and the sequence characteristics of its AAs used in enzymes and body proteins. There are eight essential AAs not manufactured in the human body: these must be imported from food intake. There are three AAs that can be manufactured – but in limited quantities. At certain times, they also become partially scarce. The other nine AAs are amply manufactured within the body. If the normal percentages held in the reserve pool of AAs in the body begin to fluctuate beyond a certain range, some AAs are dumped (differently broken or consumed) to keep the composition of the AA pool within the normal range for future protein and enzyme manufacture.

Of the AAs that get dumped in stress, tryptophan seems to be one of the most important.

However, one cannot consume this or that amino acid by itself to balance the pool, even if one knew all the intricate ramifications. *One must consume the full range of AAs to build the 'reserve pool' in due time.* The precaution one can take is to eat proteins that have these AAs in ample proportions. Some proteins, such as long-exposed meat, may become deficient in some amino acids. The best proteins are those stored in the germinating seeds of plants, such as lentils, grains, beans, and so on, and also in eggs and milk that nature provides to produce the next generation of chickens and to feed the calf.

Lentils and green beans in particular are good stores for AAs in food ingredients. They contain about 28 per cent proteins, 72 per cent complex carbohydrates, and no oil. These types of foods are by nature better stores for the provision of AAs in proportioned amounts. After all, these better choices of foods are naturally designed to procreate a perfect replica of the species concerned. The storage of a balanced amino acid composition as a life starter is an important part of the process.

Insulin-independent diabetes should be treated with an increase in water intake, exercise, and diet manipulation to provide the necessary amino acid balance for tissue repair, including brain tissue requirements. Salt regulation should also be kept in mind. Diabetes is a good example of next-generation damage that is caused by dehydration.

Whereas the onset of dehydration-induced diabetes is normally seen in the elderly and is often reversible, the more serious and structurally damaging variety of the disease is often inherited by their offspring. Juvenile diabetes will need the same approach to its early preventive treatment before permanent structural damage can take place. It should be remembered that the genetic transcription mechanism of parents – in particular the mother – if affected by amino acid pool imbalance, will be equally represented in the offspring. In effect, this is how genetic damage and inherited disorders establish. What you will read in the next few paragraphs is designed to show a representative process.

Insulin-dependent diabetes

In insulin-dependent diabetes, ability to produce insulin by pancreatic cells is lost. To control the diabetes, actual injections of insulin on a regular daily basis are essential. This condition is becoming slightly better understood.

Within the process of protein breakdown to mobilise the amino acid reserves, cortisone-releasing mechanisms also promote the secretion of a substance called IL-1 (inter-leukin). IL-1 is a neuro-transmitter. There is a magnifying effect between cortisone release mechanisms and IL-1 production; each promotes the secretion of the other. IL-1 also promotes the secretion of a subordinate substance called IL-6. Thus, continued IL-1 production will drive a simultaneous promotion of IL-6 production.

It has been shown in cell cultures that IL-6 destroys the DNA structure of insulin-producing cells. These IL-6 treated cells can not produce any more insulin. I assume (and have published this view) that continued dehydration and its unchecked disturbance of the amino acid metabolism in the body is very probably responsible for the destruction of DNA structure in the pancreas's insulin-producing beta cells. Thus, dehydration and its promotion of stress physiology may ultimately also be responsible for the emergence of insulin-dependent diabetes.

Hence, the paradigm shift can scientifically explain the role of water in disease prevention and/or cure. With strict and absolutely regular daily water intake to prevent the stresses and associated damages of dehydration, the chief conductor and supervisor of the body's well-being tryptophan and its neurotransmitter derivatives serotonin, tryptamine and melatonin will be well positioned to regulate all functions. A balanced amino acid intake in simple proteins will make sure enough of all of them is made available to the body. Regular daily walks will keep muscles well coordinated and correct any physiological processes that are established in the body as a result of anxiety and emotional 'stress'.

The above three musts are the most vital and basic anti-ageing precautions. They are essential steps to very good health and a well hydrated and healthy skin that needs water to constantly replace that which it loses to the outside environment. That is when blood vessels to the face and body will open up and provide necessary nourishment for exposed skin cells.

When the body is well hydrated, all of the physiological and hormonal prerequisites to a satisfying sex life and more-than-adequate libido will be in place. In addition, one or two glasses of water before 'the event' will help a firmer and sustained erection in men and the joys of participation in women.

CHAPTER 11

New ideas on AIDS

HIV itself is produced by a more severe
imbalance in the makeup of the
amino acid pool of the body.
It is this devastating amino
acid pool imbalance that
kills patients, not
the HIV particle.

In this section, I am sharing with you the result of many years of my
research into the physiological reasons and relationships of Acquired
Immune Deficiency Syndrome (AIDS) to metabolism disturbance
that can be caused by severe emotional and physical stress. I believe
that AIDS is not a viral disease, but a metabolic disorder precipitated
by an exaggerated way of life. It can equally be caused by severe
malnutrition in poorer and famine-stricken societies. *I know this*
view is completely against current beliefs forced by the media
presentation of a social problem, but it is the responsibility of
dedicated scientists to take it into consideration and explore all
aspects of this problem. We are only now beginning to understand
what AIDS may be. We know one thing it is not: a virus-produced
disease! At the end of this section, you will be introduced to some of
the unfolding events in AIDS research. You will also see that I have
been at the centre of the controversy.

At this point, and through the perspective of a stress-induced
metabolic system disturbance, a more accurate understanding of
AIDS may also become possible. We should not close our eyes to new
information just because we are sold on the idea that this condition is
caused by a class of viruses, conveniently called Human Immune
Deficiency Virus (HIV).

For some time now, it has been scientifically shown and recognised
that people suffering from AIDS demonstrate a marked variation

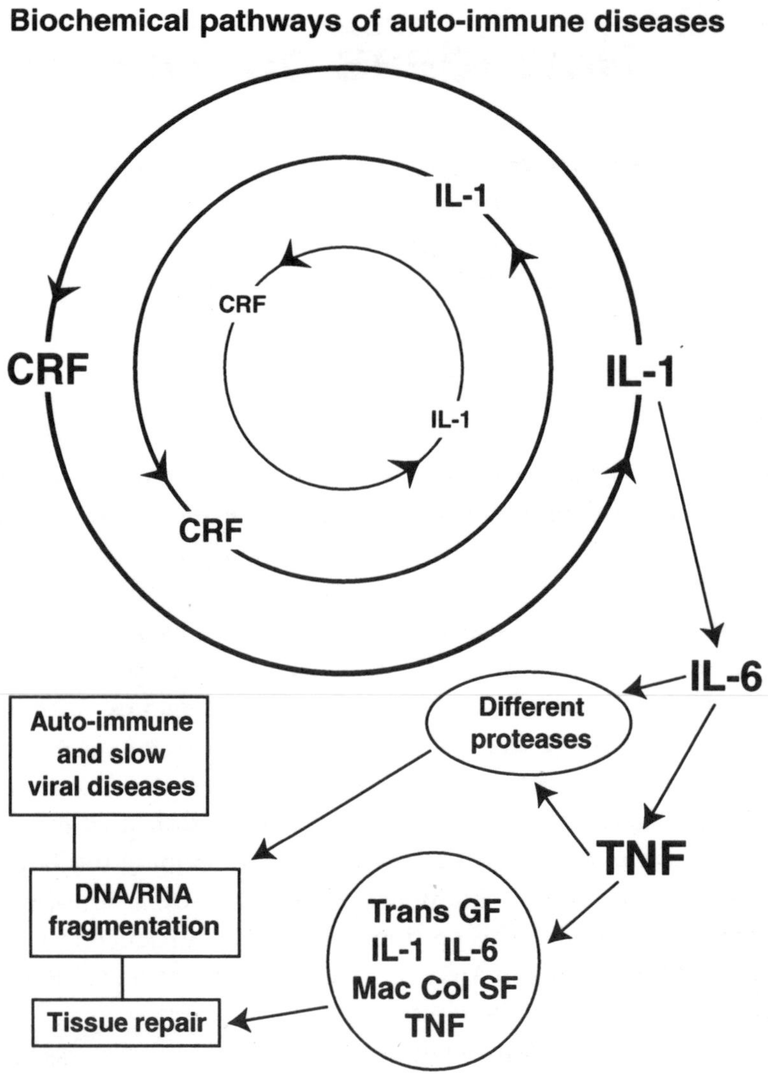

Biochemical pathways of auto-immune diseases

Key words: IL-1 = interleukin-1; IL-6 = interleukin-6; TNF = tumour necrosis factor; CRF = cortisone release factor; Trans GF = transforming growth factor; Mac Col SF = macrophage colony stimulating factor

Figure 16: The chemical model defining the main pathways to production of immune disorders. The question society must answer is this: which is more prudent – to inhibit the action of the proteases, or stop the vicious circle of CRF/IL-1?

from the normal 'amino acid pool composition' – the inventory of amino acids available in their body. *They are consistently and drastically short of methionine, cystine and cysteine – all very important amino acids. They also have a manifold rise in levels of arginine and glutamate.* This state of a very drastic amino acid imbalance seems to last for some time before the patient becomes very sick. It seems that in clinically obvious AIDS-suffering people, this pattern for amino acid composition of the body is dominant. In the section on tryptophan, it was explained that the amino acid pool composition of the body can change and become depleted if some amino acids are used up more than others.

In a series of other experiments, when IL-6 and another similar substance (TNF – tumour necrosis factor) are added to a cell culture medium that contains cells with the ability to produce the virus, particles labelled HIV are extruded. If, before the addition of IL-6 or TNF, cysteine is added to the same culture medium, HIV particles are not produced. Thus, there would seem to be a direct correlation between HIV production in AIDS and amino acid content of the virus-growing cell.

It seems that, on the face of it, AIDS patients are victims of an imbalance in their bodies' amino acid composition. If they could correct their protein metabolism, they might be able to survive, and their bodies might be able to produce sufficient resistance to fight other acute infections. After all, even for the manufacture of antibodies to defend against other bacteria, the body needs the basic amino acid ingredients in their correct proportions.

It is unfortunate that we are looking at the virus and not seeing the physiological imbalance in AIDS patients. It is also unfortunate that we do not understand the subordinate metabolic roles of IL-6 to the cortisone-releasing mechanism and IL-1 production. These agents, and others in their pack, are produced to mobilise primary raw materials from body reserves to fight stress and repair possible damages caused by having confronted any particular stressor. Their function is designed around the mechanism of breaking down proteins held in the muscles of the body and converting them to their basic amino acids for their use in the liver. So, the general direction in severe stress-damage is to mobilise the essential ingredients for their emergency re-use – a process of feeding off the body itself.

A bruised boxer or a person traumatised in an accident or after repeated surgery will depend on these physiological processes to clear the ineffective and nonviable tissue and repair, and remodel the site of damage. If the reconstruction is extensive and IL-6 and its companion TNF are involved, breakdown of DNA or RNA of the damaged and dying cells will produce exact fragments to clear the debris, very much like having to dismember the steel structure of a large building that cannot be 'bulldozed away' and has to be carried off the site, a piece at a time. This is a very well recognised process in the research of surgical wounds.

It is unfortunate that virologists are presenting the 'site clearing action' of these two agents in the body as steps in production of HIV in cell culture media. On this fragment of unconnected information is placed the whole argument that AIDS is a virus-caused disease. Why? Because a test has been designed that marks and shows the particular fragments produced by IL-6 or TNF. It seems that some of these DNA or RNA particles are labelled as HIV, which is why there are several types. It is more unfortunate that the amino acid composition of HIV itself very much resembles that of *vasopressin*. A vaccine that would arrest HIV activity will most probably arrest the activity of vasopressin. This seems to be the reason a workable vaccine against HIV has not yet been produced. Unfortunate to the extreme is the 'commercialisation of the idea' that everyone who shows a positive HIV test will soon die from AIDS, because *the anxiety of having an incurable disease could become a killer by itself*.

Without getting into the emotional side of this issue, and sticking strictly to a scientific understanding of the human body, we have to become aware of a simple fact. Tissues of the vagina and the anus and rectum are designed for different purposes. It is true both have similar sensory systems attached to a single central mechanism for the registration of pain and pleasure, but structurally they are not the same. The vagina has a thick, multilayered cell lining that, while not easily absorbing semen from inside, is designed to withstand friction and shearing force. Even here, there is a mechanism for secretion of lubricating mucus to withstand these forces. Furthermore, semen has chemical properties that will increase the thickness and resistance of the lining membrane in the vagina and the skin of the penis that becomes smeared by it.

Seminal fluid secreted with the sperm has a complex composition. It contains a chemical substance called *transglutamin-ase* (TGE). In certain circumstances, TGE binds some proteins to other proteins. It also causes some cells to die in a special way – to shrivel and not disintegrate, thus its power to produce a thickening of the vaginal wall to cope with normal male-female sex relationships. This property of semen, when introduced into the intestine, will alter the water-absorbing quality of its lining, thus the associated diarrhoea in AIDS. The semen also contains proteins with extremely strong immune suppressive properties.

It is the immune suppressive property of semen that facilitates the passage of sperm all the way up into the uterus and its tubes to fertilise the female egg. To the body, the millions of sperm that enter the uterus are invading 'foreign objects' that would be highly reactionary for the uterine wall and its tubes had they not been protected by the immune repressive properties of proteins from the semen that bathe the sperm. In order for the sperm and eventually the foetus (that has different antigenic properties from the mother's tissue) to survive during nine months of pregnancy, the mother's immune system has to be suppressed for the duration of pregnancy. It seems that something in the semen (possibly a utero-globin-like protein called SV-IV) *codes for the mother's immune suppression.* It is this immune-suppressive property of semen that ensures the survival of, initially, the sperm, and ultimately the foetus during full-term pregnancy until the birth of a living offspring. It is interesting to know that in the third trimester of pregnancy there is often a reversal of the $T_4:T_8$ ratio.

Semen in the female vagina is not absorbed. Because of the anatomical design and position of the vagina, the semen is drained. On the other hand, the rectum is lined with very thin and delicate cells. In the rectum, semen is retained and its potent physiological properties are allowed freedom of action. Within the constituents of semen, there are substances that are designed to overcome the host's immune system and force it to shut down the same way that a radar jamming device is used on board warplanes to enter enemy airspace and deliver their bombs. Thus, semen has an independent ability to shut down the immune system of its host tissue if its agents are allowed entry into the recipient's system. Because of this ability, the marker of T_4:T_8 ratio reversal is seen in homosexuals with AIDS.

With repeated secretion of semen into a male or female rectum, the immune system suppression is unavoidable not because of a 'virus', but because of chemical properties of the semen itself. Women who participate in anal sex to avoid becoming pregnant should be aware of this immune suppressive property of semen.

In addition to all of the above, the intestinal wall is not capable of withstanding the forces involved in rectal manipulation for sexual purposes. The reason such sexual manipulations become possible is because of one single fact: the intestinal tract does not have an acute pain sensory system if damaged from inside unless the damage affects the peritoneum, the thin outside cover of the gastrointestinal tract. This is amply supplied with nerves that will register pain. It is a type of 'non-adhesive' that permits various segments of the intestinal tract to glide over one another in their movements and during adaptation to the passage of food. But the rectum is not completely covered by peritoneum in the same way as the rest of the intestinal tract.

Thus, the inside lining of the rectum can become damaged without that damage registering in the same way the skin would sound the alarm when its resistance is broken. The rectum is the end part of an anatomical structure whose activity has to be performed silently. However, damage is recognised physiologically, and physiological steps for repair of the local damage will be no less vigorous.

As part and parcel of the repair mechanisms, the chemical agents TNF, IL-1, IL-6 and others in their pack will be secreted to commence the process of crisis management (Figure 16). If the damage is such that resident bacteria could also break barriers and begin increased local activity, production of these agents for crisis management will increase. (It has been shown experimentally that AIDS patients have markedly increased levels of IL-6 and TNF in their blood.) This raised

IL-6, as it was explained in the section on diabetes, will also destroy the insulin-producing cells in the pancreas. Hence, a simple explanation for diabetes seen in the advanced stages of full-blown AIDS.

These agents function very much like a team of specialist salvage workers that go to a site after an earthquake. One group would clear the debris; others would bring survival supplies for those caught in the area who cannot be relocated; another would begin to restore power, water, and telephone services, and so on. In the everyday life of a city, all these processes take place, and they are carried out by people and machines. In the human body, the same processes occur. The agents that perform these necessary functions are hormones and their subordinate enzyme systems. The principle is the same. Each cell has a personality and needs to survive on the spot if it can be repaired. Only the dead or irreparably damaged cells will have to be dismembered and cleared away.

In rectal manipulation, should there be more than routine wear and tear, these same agents become operatives for its repair. It will take time to reproduce the original 'blueprint' and fully restore local tissues. Should there be a recurrence of the injury, on top of a tissue that is already weak, more forceful presence of these local repair agents will be called for. There may come a time when these hormones and their subordinate operators will be *permanently* commissioned and their presence in the blood circulation will become measurable. Since the relationship and significance of their increased presence for the repair of the 'unsensed' local damage in the rectum is not appreciated – and furthermore, the rationale of their activity not recognised – part of their mechanism of function is highlighted and labelled as the causative factor for the physiological upheaval that is conveniently labelled as 'AIDS' for public consumption.

In laboratory research, it has been shown that cysteine prevents the production of HIV in cultured cells. Other laboratory research has shown that AIDS patients are short of cysteine and its precursor cystine. In two simple-to-understand experiments, a metabolic basis to the development of the disease has been clearly demonstrated. If the cells that are sufficiently abnormal to produce HIV are given *cysteine*, their abnormality is corrected and they do not produce the

HIV. All we need to know now is how these AIDS patients became cysteine-deficient. We should commence the research of this phenomenon and not sidetrack AIDS research into a dead end by making a jump of faith and assuming it to be virus-produced.

In my opinion, it seems the 'HIV test' highlights the presence of a fragment of DNA or RNA of a damaged cell – it indicates a process of cell nucleus breakdown. It could be produced by many other factors, one of them *cysteine and zinc* deficiency, particularly in people from underdeveloped and poorer countries. It is also possible that it is caused as a result of persistent and increasingly severe local damage in the rectum, producing a long-term run on the body's protein reserves. This test by itself is not an accurate indicator of the presence of an agent that causes the disease. *The HIV itself is produced by a more severe imbalance in the makeup of the amino acid pool of the body. It is this devastating amino acid pool imbalance that kills patients, not the HIV particle.*

As soon as this statement is made, questions pop up in the minds of people who have had to focus on HIV spread through blood. *It is true that the blood may contain the released HIV particles, but this blood also contains many other hormones and transmitters – some of which are not yet known. One cannot assume AIDS to be caused by HIV unless physiological effects of the various other components in the serum or blood are known.*

As a hypothetical example, Sir Peter Medawar, FRS, a Nobel laureate and president of the Royal Society in England expressed the opinion that there are certain human genes that, once triggered, programme the death of the individual. In other words, even death is an orderly and controlled phenomenon. The question arises as to whether people who lose fine gender definition and become disinterested in nature's normal procreation programme are more susceptible to the activation of the genes that can cause their early demise.

In a series of very significant experiments scientists Brodish and Lymangrove have shown that 'stressed intestines' produce a local hormone that has a very strong and long-lasting activity. Experiments have shown TCRF to be stronger than normal cortisone-releasing mechanisms . This hormone could be transfused in the serum from one animal to another. It stays in the new animal for some time and has exactly the same cortisone-releasing activity.

Cortisone-release mechanisms, at certain levels, will result in the production of some nucleus breakdown and DNA fragmentation similar to HIV particle formation. Again, this is a metabolic disorder even if the tests are perceived to represent HIV particle formation.

We should understand that all manufacturing processes in the cells of the body are taking place in a fluid medium; parts can float away unless an anchoring system is in place. A very important point that needs clarification is the fact that many units of cysteine are involved in the formation of a type of anchoring 'rope' that has *zinc hooks* attached to a number of cysteines. These keep the DNA assembly line in position and prevent the drift of its segments, much like washing lines with their hooks for open-air drying of clothes. *The sex hormone receptor's structure formation and function in men and women depends very strongly on the presence of these zinc and cysteine 'fingers'.* Thus, the deficiency of cysteine in the bodies of those with AIDS could have a far greater significance than may initially be apparent. Could the loss of gender dominance in either sex be initially caused by changes in the amino acid pool composition of the body, with *'comparative'* cysteine, and possibly zinc, deficiency at the top of the list? This is a strong possibility.

One should be aware that when the correct mix of amino acids to procreate a normal offspring is not available to the body, its direct impact is on sex hormones and their receptors. One must assume they are 'decommissioned' lest the natural design of the species gets drastically changed. It should be remembered the natural design to sexuality is its outcome of procreation and rearing of offspring. The associated addictive 'high' is the driving force behind the design.

Now comes a social dilemma! Homosexuality may lead to a much faster eradication from nature's inventory of its creations.

By joining so many disease conditions by the acronym of AIDS, and by getting the public to think of AIDS as a single disease produced by a slow virus, my colleagues in this branch of research are doing a disservice to mankind. They sharply deviate from the truth and in the process secure more research funds, sell more test kits and promote the sale of poisonous chemicals that accelerate the deterioration of the health of those so treated.

Another question that might be asked concerns the relationship of intravenous morphine and heroin use to the production of AIDS. The answer may possibly be found in chemical properties of these substances on body physiology. Morphine-like substances register their effect through the nerve system, which sends messages around by the use of serotonin as its neurotransmitter agent. This nerve system and morphine-like substances are able to alter the metabolic pattern of the body. Endorphins, the natural morphines of the body, not only suppress pain sensation and produce euphoria, they also alter the level of hunger sensation.

Furthermore, those who use these drugs on a regular basis are highly stressed people, either by the initial reason that forced them to take drugs, or by the difficulty of getting a regular supply. In any event, stress physiology sets in and, because of altered metabolism, not enough of the body's daily needs will be met. When morphine or heroin is used, sensations of hunger and thirst are also suppressed and the body begins to feed off itself. In countries where people used to smoke opium, a great number of these people eventually died of lung infections – *exactly what is now blamed on the virus and contaminated needles.*

It is also important to know there is a time gap of many years between recognition of 'HIV' in the body and production of clinical symptoms of immune suppression. *I can assure you, the amino acid imbalance during this time gap becomes a far more potent killer than the 'virus of AIDS'.* At the beginning, the body begins to produce antibodies to the virus. It is only after some time that production of all antibodies becomes insufficient and ineffective. *We should not forget that a balanced and well proportioned amino acid pool composition in the body is essential for antibody production.*

One terrible aspect of AIDS is the cruelty with which it affects babies born to mothers who are HIV positive. It should be clear that if the mother is deficient in certain amino acids in her body, she is not able to provide the baby with the correct range of amino acids for its normal development. Should the mother be even minimally deficient in her methionine, cystine, cysteine, tryptophan and others, the baby is bound to be short of these same elements that will possibly predispose to DNA fragmentation in the process of cell development, particularly in the breast-feeding phase.

Unfolding events in AIDS research

As the first edition of this book was being written, a group of AIDS research scientists from Europe and America gathered in Holland in May 1992 to begin a movement against the established and protected thinking on AIDS as a viral disease. As reported in the *Sunday Times* of 26 April 1992, two interesting members of this group were France's Professor Luc Montagnier and Professor Duesberg from America.

Professor Luc Montagnier of the Pasteur Institute is the original discoverer of the virus that was later labelled as HIV. He isolated the virus that was supposed to have inhibited the immune system. He sent samples to Robert Gallo in America, who was also working on a method for isolation and testing an AIDS virus. Dr Gallo later applied for a patent on a test kit. The French started legal proceedings to claim their rights for the discovery of the virus. Eventually, and after much legal hassle, the two parties agreed to share a portion of the proceeds from the marketing of the test kit. The rest of the proceeds were to be devoted to further research of AIDS. But the French forced further investigations into allegations of scientific impropriety. After more thorough scrutiny, it was conceded that Dr Gallo had initially used the French sample for his patent.

Professor Montagnier seemed to have reversed his original views and claimed the virus was not of primary importance in AIDS. The newspaper interview indicated that the professor accepted that AIDS might have other causes. He seemed to acknowledge the possible existence of AIDS even without the presence of HIV. The professor must have found compelling arguments that deny HIV as the culprit and the single cause of all the group of diseases classified under AIDS. A drastic change took place in Professor Montagnier's thinking.

Professor Duesberg, who had researched the actual composition of the virus, at the same time as others were believing in its disease-producing properties, announced the virus incapable of causing

AIDS. There were many debates, but his arguments did not cut any ice with the established group busy with AIDS viral research in America and in Europe. He could not offer an alternative scientific explanation on the cause of the diseases grouped together under AIDS other than saying the disease is not caused by a virus. The researchers in this field were looking for plausible scientific ideas to find a solution to the problem. A statement to the effect that AIDS is not a viral disease was not enough. Scientific reasons which point in another direction should have accompanied the negation of HIV as the cause of the disease.

I wrote to Dr Manfred Eigen, an eminent DNA research scientist from the Max-Planck Institute in Germany, on 25 September 1989 and in defence of Duesberg sent him two of my articles presenting most of the views that were published in the Foundation for the Simple in Medicine's Special AIDS Issue. Dr Eigen had published an account of discussions between AIDS virus advocates and Duesberg in *Natur Wissenschaften*. It seems Dr Eigen was not convinced by Professor Duesberg's views and had taken the side of the opposition. A few months later, Dr Eigen sent me a letter that showed he realised another plausible scientific view on the cause of AIDS did exist.

So, all of a sudden in 1992 a new surge of activity with an alternative view of AIDS had gathered momentum with both Professors Montagnier and Duesberg as leaders in the field.

In 1989 I had sent these researchers a copy of our Special AIDS Issue of *Science In Medicine Simplified* (*SMS*) from the Foundation, in the same way the Foundation freely shares its views with most top researchers (a copy of the letter to Manfred Eigen was also sent to Professor Duesberg). This special AIDS volume was also sent to many medical libraries at universities engaged in AIDS research. The detailed articles presented scientific explanations from which a synopsis has been given in the preceding paragraphs.

In my article on the neurotransmitter histamine, first presented briefly at the 3rd Interscience World Conference on Inflammation in 1989 and later published in 1990, I also explained the immune suppressive actions of many of the chemical agents that are generated as a result of stress in the human body. In this extensively distributed article I discussed some aspects of AIDS as a severe stress-induced 'system disturbance', opposing the current view that it is caused by a single particle, a virus.

This issue of *SMS* was also extensively distributed. Copies of the 1989 Special AIDS Issue and 1990 issue of *SMS* were also sent to Professor Philippe Lazar, the Director General of INSERM in France, the French equivalent of the National Institute of Health (NIH) in America. He was asked to make the information available to other interested scientists at INSERM.

My research was progressing at the same time as new information on the critical roles of cysteine in the manufacture of some DNA materials became available and published. It became completely clear and obvious to me that AIDS was a metabolic disorder and the DNA/RNA fragments classified as the different viruses of AIDS were themselves a product of cysteine shortage in the body. With infinitely more detail than has been presented in this section, my most recent article of that period, 'AIDS: The Dead-End of Virus Aetiology' was published in the 1991 issue of *SMS* and distributed to many other scientists engaged in this field of research.

It is the moral obligation of any dedicated scientist to share his or her new information with others engaged in the research of a common topic, even before the subject is presented in scientific journals. It is also a moral obligation of those who receive the information to give credit to the person who has generated and shared the information.

A news headline in *Le Monde* of 9 August 1991 reflected a heated fight between Bruno Durieux, the Minister of Health of France and Professor Albert German, President of the National Academy of Pharmacy of France. The minister had demanded the dismissal of the professor. The professor had, in an address, given the opinion that AIDS is caused as a result of a particular life style. The professor's opinion had become a hot issue among the different social groups, thus the wrath of the minister and the demand for his dismissal. No occasion lends itself better to the introduction of an explosive opinion than adding it as fuel to an already established quarrel. The following letter was sent to M. Bruno Durieux, Minister of Health of France, with a copy to Professor German.

FOUNDATION FOR THE SIMPLE IN MEDICINE
A MEDICAL RESEARCH INSTITUTION
P.O. BOX 3267 FALLS CHURCH VA 22043 U.S.A.

Exc. M. Bruno Durieux
Minister of Health
1 Place de Fontenoy
75350 Paris 07-S.P.
6 September 1991

Excellence,
I have been exposed to the topic of your discussion about the views of Professor Albert German on AIDS, reflected in Le Monde, *9 August 1991. I thought it my responsibility to bring to your attention the final result of our very extensive research into the aetiology of AIDS. Our research seems to produce physiologic/ metabolic explanations that support the views of Professor German. I have pleasure in enclosing a copy of our recent article, 'AIDS: The Dead-End of Virus Aetiology'. The article explains details that have been ignored by those who wish to force a solution to the problem through viral research – a total waste of public funds. You are welcome to have the article photocopied and reviewed by any number of your scientists who do not demonstrate a blind bias toward viral research. If more information is needed, please do not hesitate to contact me.*
Sincerely,
F. Batmanghelidj, MD

Enclosure: Article, AIDS: The Dead-End of Virus Aetiology.
Copy, Professor Albert German.

I hope the free sharing of my researched views on AIDS has in some way been instrumental in getting others to think about the relationship of this disease condition to an abnormal physiology that becomes established as a result of 'stresses associated with a particular life style' or 'severe malnutrition in less fortunate societies'. The children in Romania that were the subject of many television programmes most probably did not get AIDS from blood contamination; they more than likely developed AIDS as a result of malnutrition.

Another point that needs to be discussed is the value of the AIDS test as an indicator of a disease in the process of development. Although everyone is led to believe this is valid, it is in my opinion an erroneous representation of a different truth. All the test shows is that the body has come across this antigenic particle and registered its structure. It also means the body has kept the existence of this particle/virus in its memory-bank to manufacture a suitable defence mechanism against the 'foreign particle', not necessarily a particle from outside but one the body itself should not make – a form of quality control at the 'DNA assembly line'. So ultimately this test is an indicator of a body's amino acid metabolism disturbance, and not an indicator of a loose killer virus in the body. *The number of test positive cases who become HIV negative are too many to be ignored.*

It has been shown in laboratory experiments that if cysteine is added to a culture medium that is growing cells for virus production, these cells will not manufacture the 'virus'. In a medium with sufficient cysteine, it will not be possible to harvest the virus. This test presents the clear conclusion that the AIDS test is only an indicator of an on-going amino acid imbalance in the body. It is important to remember that if the level of one amino acid in the body is not enough, then a drastic imbalance in the percentage composition of the other amino acids also will exist.

These new ideas on AIDS are presented here to indicate that a metabolic approach to dealing with this social problem will produce more satisfactory and quicker results, whilst possibly boosting the expressions of normal gender definition.

An easy way to stop muscle breakdown is by an intelligent adjustment of the daily water intake and by eating a balanced high-protein diet.

Take a look at Edward Dippre's letter overleaf. As you can see, water and some salt intake have reversed muscle breakdown in a dehydration-produced 'disease' condition. Because the cause was not known, the problem was labelled 'muscular dystrophy'.

217 North Street
West Pittston, Pa. 18643
March 15, 1995

Dear Dr Batmanghelidj,
Around November 1 my legs were giving out. They became black
and blue from my knees to my thighs, and very painful. I went to the
doctor and he told me that my muscle enzymes were at 660 and
normal was 90. Then I went to another doctor and he said I had
muscular dystrophy.

I started talking to Dr Batmanghelidj who told me to start
drinking two quarts of water daily. I have been, I feel much better,
and all symptoms disappeared in two months. I also use sea salt
liberally with all my meals.

I went back to the doctor and had additional bloodwork done.
The enzyme levels in my muscles were back to normal, and the
doctor couldn't understand how it was possible.

As of this date I am free of all discomfort and symptoms. I also
have more energy and better health than I can remember for a
long time.
Sincerely,
Edward Dippre

Enhancing daily exercise and physical activity force the body into
a physiological programme to build up its muscles instead of breaking
them into their amino acid components to feed the rest of the body.
You need to realise the human body is designed to defend itself
against all types of infections. It survived fast acting viruses such as
smallpox, measles, polio, and others during its development. It
generally takes the body about nine days to mount an effective
defence against even fast viruses. If the body can survive fast viruses,
surely it must be more than capable of defending itself against slow-
growing viruses?

All that we need to understand is how to make the body stronger
and stop actions that would make it vulnerable.

CHAPTER 12

The simplest of treatments in medicine

'You cannot by reasoning correct a man of ill opinion which by reasoning he never acquired.'
Francis Bacon

Your body needs an *absolute minimum* of six to eight 8-ounce glasses of water per day.

Alcohol, coffee, tea, and caffeine-containing beverages don't count as water.

The best times to drink water (clinically observed in peptic ulcer disease) are: one glass one half hour before taking food – breakfast, lunch, and dinner – and a similar amount two and a half hours after each meal. This is the very minimum amount of water your body needs. For the sake of not short-changing your body, two more glasses of water should be taken around the heaviest meal or before going to bed.

Thirst should be satisfied at all times. With increase in water intake, the thirst mechanism becomes more efficient. Your body might then ask you to drink more than the above minimum.

Adjusting water intake to mealtimes prevents the blood from becoming concentrated as a result of food intake. When the blood becomes concentrated, it draws water from the cells around it.

Water is the cheapest form of medicine to a dehydrated body. As simply as dehydration will in time produce the major diseases we are confronting now, a well regulated and constantly alert attention to daily water intake will help to prevent the emergence of most of the major diseases we have come to fear in our modern society.

William Gray's letter is introduced here in this chapter as a telling example of how water is a better medication for the treatment of so many differently labelled complications of chronic dehydration. As you will see, Mr Gray is a highly intelligent person. His observations provide a great deal of insight into the possible complications of chronic dehydration in the human body.

It is for this reason that I selected this section of the book in which to present his observations. My hope is to impress upon your mind a simple fact. There is more natural magic in a glassful of water than any medication you are brainwashed into using for treatment of conditions I have talked about in this book. And I do not sell water!

From: William E Gray (Bill)
411 Ayrhill Avenue
Vienna, VA 22180
11 - 2 - 94
703 - 938 - 6330

To: Dr Batmanghelidj
2146 Kings Garden Way
Falls Church, VA 22043

It has been one year since I first read your book, which was given to me as a present by Marcel Thevoz. Since then my health has improved significantly. I am now 52 and in excellent health. This was not the case before your book and Marcel's kindness inspired me to make water an integral part of my life.

To most people I was successful and in excellent health – normal weight, unusual strength and endurance, above average at sports, with an excellent diet (a lot of fresh vegetables and whole grains and very little meat, animal products or processed food). Yet my list of complaints stretches over the last fifty years and includes: duodenal ulcer (age 19), indigestion, colon and elimination problems (age 19 to 51), food allergies (age 12 to 17), chronic sinus infection (age 5 to 51), chronic and acute back problems (age 13 through age 51), emotional illness and mental confusion (age 6 to age 51).

These problems were even more bewildering and confusing

because I am intelligent, educated and motivated to find solutions to problems.

I have been searching for answers to these problems for 35 years. I have looked for answers in: diet, diet supplementation, exercise, yoga, meditation, Traditional Religion, spiritual practices, Acupuncture, traditional medicine, Chiropractic, Massage, Raki, Polarity Balancing, 12 Step programs, and self improvement books and courses, such as Est and the Hoffman Quadrinity Process.

I had, of course, read many times about the importance of drinking plenty of water. I even invested in a reverse osmosis water filter six years ago, hoping that the improved taste of the water would motivate me to drink more water. In spite of this, I never gave water therapy a fair chance. Until I read your book, other beverages always looked better to me, particularly tea and coffee.

At the time I read your book I had a chronic nerve injury in my upper back that intermittently prevented me from playing golf or racket ball for a period of two years. My arm strength was a third of what it had been only two years previously. I was at a low point in my life physically and mentally.

I have never been drunk in my life or smoked more than five cigarettes in a day. At the time I was not smoking or drinking alcohol. Yet I found myself obsessed with thoughts of caffeine, smoking and drinking. Although I have been a frequent visitor at Chiropractic, Osteopathic and Massage therapists, I had not needed to visit a medical doctor for 15 years. In my desperation I went to an MD who prescribed an anti-stress medication, a pain reliever, and a muscle relaxant. I took the prescribed doses and fell into a semi-coma for 16 hours, and discontinued the medication. A few weeks later Marcel came to my home for dinner and gave me your book.

Within one week of adding two to three quarts of water to my diet noticed I that:

The pain from the nerve injury went away and I was able to begin exercising.

I had much less indigestion and gas.

My urges and compulsive behaviour lessened substantially or vanished. I no longer had to fight the urge to smoke, drink, stuff myself or use excessive caffeine.

My energy levels improved.

My thinking and work improved.

Please feel free to use me as a reference. I am happy to talk to anyone about water at any time.

William E Gray

Ordinary tap water, unless there is proof of its being contaminated with chemicals and heavy metals such as lead, is a good source of supply. Tap water has the protection of chlorine as a bacteria-killing agent. The bottled water in supermarkets is said to be sterilised by the addition of ozone at the time of bottling. Ozone, of 'super oxygen', seems to have a bacteria-killing property. If used in time, bottled water can serve as an alternative source of supply. If you are not sure whether your water source is contaminated or contains impurities not safe to drink, save yourself from this anxiety by installing a small filtration unit on your kitchen tap. There are very effective carbon or ceramic filter units that can save you from the hassle of buying and carrying water from stores every day.

Eventually, filtration of water at point of use will become standard practice in advanced societies that have a tendency to pollute drinking water. With the present decline in the fortunes of the municipalities, delivering quality drinking water in their pipe systems will at some point become prohibitively expensive. It won't make economic sense to deliver high quality water for use in washing and gardening.

If one develops a taste for other than tap water and runs out of supplies at home, the body may be forced to go without water just because of a dislike of the taste of tap water: a self-imposed preference. Usually, the 'bad taste' is attributed to dissolved chlorine in the water. Most sales agents who wish to sell water purifiers make issue of the fact that tap water contains chlorine. They also point to calcium dissolved in the water, often termed 'hard water'.

However, if we fill an open-top jug with water and let it stand in the refrigerator or on the kitchen counter, chlorine that is dissolved in the water will evaporate and the smell of it will also disappear. The water will become sweet and very easily palatable. This is how all restaurants serve water – out of a well-iced jug that was filled some time before its use.

As for the calcium in water, unless the water is truly and *heavily* calcium-laden, its use is perfectly safe. Not only is it safe, it is a cheap source of calcium needed by the body. Calcium is already dissolved in the water and one does not need to go to the pharmacy to buy calcium tablets to take as a preventive measure against the onset of osteoporosis we see in the elderly.

How and when do you think osteoporosis begins? Actually, many years before it is recognised. When hydroelectric energy stores become depleted on and off, energy stored in the bondage of calcium to calcium in the cells and eventually in the bones is used. When one molecule of calcium becomes separated from another molecule of calcium, one unit of ATP is also released. ATP is one unit of exchangeable energy. The loose calcium is now available to be shed. When water and calcium are taken in their natural forms, the emergency need for the release of energy stored in calcium bondage is decreased. This is why bones are a great source of reserved energy. The body is able to tap into this reservoir of energy.

In any case, even heavily-dissolved calcium in the water will most probably be without adverse effects. It seems the body possesses a most delicate need-regulated mechanism for absorption of elements from the gastrointestinal tract. Most probably, not all the calcium dissolved in even very hard water enters the system.

A recent study (in another country and in a region with only very hard water available for consumption) has shown the calcium-laden water consumed did not produce any adverse effects on the people who did not avoid drinking the water.

To prevent disease, one does not actually need to stick to strict diet manipulation to control this or that clinical condition as long as water intake precedes food intake. However, one word of advice is to limit fatty and fried foods. Fats get converted to fatty acids and circulate in the blood. Fatty acids will replace tryptophan that is attached to the albumin to be stored and protected while being circulated around in the blood.

The liver will attack and destroy freed tryptophan if its free form in circulation is more than 20 per cent of its total content. In due time, excess fatty food will therefore deplete the body's tryptophan reserves. This is one of the most important reasons why fatty foods are not good for health.

At the same time, not all fatty acids are bad for the body. In fact, there are at least two essential fatty acids that the body needs all the time and cannot manufacture. They are: alpha-linolenic acid (LNA), known as Omega 3 oil, and linoleic acid (LA), known as Omega 6 oil. These fatty acids are needed for the manufacture of cell membranes, hormones and nerve coverings in the body.

Although other fats that enter the body are used for their energy content, O-3 and O-6 are saved and used only for the manufacture of hormones and in the structure of all of the membranes inside and covering the cell. In treatment of those diseases that result from damage to the nerve covering, the regular intake of these essential fatty acids is a must.

The richest source of O-3 is flax seed, from which flax oil is extracted and sold on the market. Flax oil also contains some O-6 in its composition. The richest sources of O-6 are safflower and sunflower oils. Flax oil is already on the market. Dr Udo Erasmus, author of the book *Fats That Kill, Fats That Heal,* based on many years of research, has developed a special mix of the essential oils the body needs for its different manufacturing programmes. Udo's Choice contains: flax oil, sunflower oil, sesame oil, rice germ oil, wheat germ oil, oat germ oil, lecithin, vitamin E, and some special triglycerides. Taking six to eight grammes (a spoonful) of this mix each day should provide all the essential fatty acids that the body needs. For more information on oils, read Dr Erasmus's book.

Loss of hair, sterility, weakness, impaired vision, growth retardation, eczema, liver damage, kidney damage, and other degenerative conditions may also be associated with essential fatty acid deficiency in the body.

Easing sleeping: Do you have difficulty in sleeping at night? Try drinking a glass of water and then putting a pinch of salt on your tongue. My personal experience and observation of others have shown that one begins falling asleep within a few minutes. In my estimation, this combination alters the rate of electrical discharge in the brain and induces sleep. Remember not to touch the palate with the salt because that may cause irritation. A cup of yoghurt at night before going to sleep will also help. It works as if you have taken a sleeping pill.

Preventing fainting: If you are susceptible to feeling faint after a shower, recognise that the water reserves of your body are not enough to reach your brain when the blood vessels in the skin open up because of the heat from the hot shower. Always drink water before going under the shower. Drink more water and increase your salt intake if you feel faint when you stand up.

Preventing heart attack: A friend of mine was hospitalised after a heart attack followed by heart arrest. He had collapsed in his office and had to be resuscitated to begin breathing again. He now has neurological complications because no oxygen had reached his brain when his heart stopped beating. For a number of days prior to his attack, he had niggly chest pains that projected into his left arm. He paid no attention to these, thinking they would go away. His mistake has landed him and his family in considerable emotional and post-stroke nursing problems. If he had learned that anginal pain that projects into the arm is a late complication of chronic dehydration, and if he had started increasing his daily water intake in response, he probably would not have suffered from such catastrophic and irreversible damage.

Please, for the sake of those who love and care for you, remember to increase your daily water intake if you are experiencing anginal pain. You should also begin to exercise and take regular walks.

Healthy urine: Urine should, ideally, be almost colourless to light yellow. If it begins to become dark yellow, or even orange, in colour, you are becoming dehydrated. This means that the kidneys are working hard to get rid of toxins in the body in very concentrated urine. Dark-coloured urine is a strong sign of dehydration.

Hopes for curing already-established disease

We have thus far discussed disease *prevention*. I have shared with you a scientific and researched opinion, based on clinical observations, and a list of diseases that seem to arise from chronic dehydration. My aim is to arm you for future prevention of disease.

However, you might already be suffering from the adverse effects of dehydration and wish to reverse the tide of events that have already taken place. Let us hope that you are still at a stage where some reversal of the disease process can be hoped for. Of course, nothing can be promised. All we can do is hope that we can establish a correction pattern.

Do not forget that, at each phase of life, our body is the product of a time-operated series of chemical interactions. Armed with correct knowledge, it might be possible to reverse some reactions. *First and foremost, do not imagine you can reverse the situation if you now 'drown' yourself in water.* The cells of the body are like sponges; it takes some time before they become better hydrated. Also do not forget that some of them make their membranes less permissive of water diffusion in or out.

The first place to show signs of being 'over-watered' is the lungs, if your kidneys do not filter the excess water. If your kidneys are not damaged as a result of long-standing and expanding dehydration resulting from the loss of thirst sensation, then you can feel safe and drink the specified amount.

If your kidneys have also suffered from the need to concentrate and pass the toxic chemicals that keep building up within the body in long-endured and increasing dehydration, then you have to be very cautious. You must also be under medication and professional supervision. You cannot just cut your medication and begin drinking water in place of these chemical manipulators of the body chemistry. You should, for a few days, assess exactly the quantity of water you normally drink and the amount of urine you pass. Now begin adding one or two glasses of water a day to the amount you usually drink. Also measure the quantity of urine you pass. If the amount of urine you pass begins to increase, then you can also increase the water you take. If you are on diuretics, remember that water is the best natural diuretic if the kidneys are functioning normally. *In my opinion, it is ignorance-based 'science' to prescribe the intake of diuretics in place of increasing water intake, if the kidneys of a patient are capable of producing urine.*

The vogue in medical practice has become the spontaneous and indiscriminate use of diuretics, calcium blockers, beta blockers, and anti-cholesterol medications in the type of patients exemplified by Mr John Fox (see pages 91–92). Why? Simply because the 'science' of medicine has expanded on a hopelessly erroneous paradigm. The very foundation of 'knowledge' on which medical practice of today is staking its credibility and licence to practise is in error, and ignorant of water metabolism disturbance as a possible cause of disease emergence in the human body.

That is how I was taught medicine before I discovered *my own ignorance.* After reading my book, Dr Julian Whitaker in the October 1994 edition of his newsletter, *Health and Healing,* distributed to 550,000 people, described his own similar experience. He stated: 'In medical school I learned that water was unimportant to the body. Water was inactive, simply along for the ride.' I am told that he is advising those who attend his clinic about chronic dehydration. Your local doctor has the same basis of wrong education about the human body and its calls for water. Now that you know better, tell him where he has gone wrong in your case. Ask him to supervise your condition when you begin to adjust your daily water intake and your diet. If he or she is unfamiliar with what you are talking about, share the information you have acquired on the problems associated with long-standing chronic dehydration of the body.

The body constantly strives to retain salt to keep water inside the system. It takes a gradual increase in urine to pass out excess salt. Water will do this if the intake is increased very gradually. *When urine formation is reduced and some oedema (swelling) of the legs and eyelids are present, increased water intake should be proportionate to increased urine production.*

As puffiness of the eyes and swelling of the ankles begin to show signs of reducing, then water intake can be increased. Inadvertent collection of water in the lungs must be avoided. That is why I insist on an accurate measurement of fluid intake and urine output if you wish to test the effect of increasing your daily water intake and reducing your coffee and tea intake.

A salt-free diet is utterly stupid

Salt is an essential ingredient of the body. In their order of importance, oxygen, water, salt and potassium are the primary elements for the survival of the human body. Pliny, around A D 75, called salt *'foremost among human remedies'.* He was right, because about 27 per cent of the salt content of the body is stored in the bones as crystals. It is said that salt crystals naturally make bones hard. Thus salt deficiency in the body could be responsible for the development of osteoporosis, because salt is taken out of the bones to maintain its vital normal levels in the blood.

Low salt intake will contribute to acidity build-up in some cells. High cell acidity can damage DNA structure and be the initiating mechanism for cancer formation in some cells. Experiments have shown that quite a number of cancer patients show low salt levels.

Let me repeat: when the body begins to collect salt, it is doing so to keep water in the body. From this 'oedema fluid', it can filter some of its water and flush it through the cell membrane into some of the cells. The principle is the same as that in the water purification process used in reverse osmosis plants to manufacture drinking water for communities without direct access to fresh water. That is why the rise in blood pressure to build a filtration force is necessary.

It is important to be alert to loss of salt from the body when water intake is increased and salt intake is not. After a few days of taking six or eight or ten glasses of water a day, you should begin to think of *adding some salt* to your diet. If you begin to feel muscle cramps at night, remember you are becoming salt-deficient. *Cramps in unexercised muscles most often mean salt shortage in the body.* Also, dizziness and feeling faint may be indicators of salt and water shortage in the body. If such occasions arise, *you should also begin to increase your vitamin and mineral intake, particularly if you are dieting to lose weight and are not including vegetables and fruits with water-soluble vitamin and mineral content.*

I have developed a rule of thumb for daily salt intake. For every ten glasses of water (about 2 quarts/4 litres), one should add to the diet about half of a teaspoon of salt per day. An average teaspoon can contain 6 grammes of salt. Half of a teaspoon is about 3 grammes of salt. Of course, you should make sure that your kidneys are producing urine. Otherwise the body will swell up. If you sense your skin and ankles are beginning to swell, do not panic. Reduce salt intake for a few days, but increase your water intake until the swelling in the legs has disappeared.

You should also increase your exercise: muscle activity will draw the excess fluid into the blood circulation and some salt is then lost in perspiration and urine. But you should be careful not to sit or stand in one position for too long.

Carrots (for their beta-carotene content) are an essential dietary requirement. Beta-carotene is a precursor for vitamin A and is absolutely essential for liver metabolism, as well as being needed by the eyes.

Some orange juice for its potassium content should also be added to the fluid intake of the body. But please remember that more is not better. Too much orange juice will cause problems of its own. If the body is overloaded with potassium, histamine production in the body will increase.

I have helped people get rid of long-standing asthma attacks by a simple piece of advice: they were asked to limit their orange juice intake to one, at most two, glasses a day – replacing the rest of the daily juice intake by water.

The vast majority of very frequently used medications are either directly or indirectly strong antihistamines. The strongest variety is used in psychiatry, for patients with depression. Many antidepressant drugs on the market are antihistamines, to the extent that some gastroenterologists actually use these drugs for the treatment of ulcer patients because they are cheaper. There are many on the market and, because of competition, their prices are lower than the traditional H_2 blocking agents.

This information is given to indicate that the pharmaceutical industry appreciates the significance of histamine activity in the human body. They are not interested in informing us of the role of histamine in water regulation of the body; they are interested in marketing their products. The next time your physician prescribes a medication, ask if it has any antihistamine activity. *Antihistamine medications strongly affect the immune systems of the body at the level of the bone marrow.*

The health care system and our responsibilities

If you have suffered because of the application of medical ignorance to your body's earlier calls for water, it becomes the responsibility of your attending doctor to supervise your return to health by tailing off the chemicals used to treat the chronic dehydration in your body. You should make sure your doctor becomes aware of the information on water metabolism, and your body's other call signals for water, when dehydration begins to alter the physiology of your body. Your doctor is responsible to you and, as your physician, he needs to become informed.

It is *your* responsibility to help your doctor become aware of the paradigm shift. It is your responsibility to help change the health care system to work for *you* and not the commercial and political aims of its administrators.

It may become necessary to pass legislation to ensure exclusion of dehydration as a causative factor in disease conditions before any pharmaceutical or invasive procedures are undertaken. Evaluation of drugs for ultimate use in treatment procedures should be carried out only after patients are fully hydrated and several days have elapsed before starting the test.

After all, water used in taking a pill is immediately more effective in a dehydrated person than the chemical composition of the pill! I have explained that the placebo effect seen in drug trials is most probably the result of some correction for unrecognised dehydration contributing to the disease production. You are now in the 'arena'. Please try to use the knowledge you have gained from this book and any consequent practical experience for the benefit of mankind, to attempt to bring into the practice of medicine the paradigm shift on water metabolism of the body.

Cost savings to the nation

When the paradigm change in medicine is fully adopted and practised, it will save a large portion of the vast and unnecessary health care costs and expenditure by society. Hypertension and its associated cardiovascular disorders are costing the USA over 100 billion dollars a year. Back pain translates into an 80-billion-dollar-a-year loss to society. Rheumatoid joint disease is affecting 20 million elderly people and is costing the USA many tens of billions of dollars annually, to name but a *few* disabling conditions.

A simple correction of this long-standing scientific mistake can reverse the budget deficit of this nation. In any event, *the paradigm shift will also produce a much healthier society.* It is estimated that the runaway cost of health care in this society will increase to 28 per cent of the gross national product by the year 2010. Even with such a rise in expenditure, 50 million people in the USA will not be able to afford to pay the rising costs of health insurance and will be deprived of adequate coverage. *The paradigm shift will reverse this 'no solution in sight' spiralling trend in health care costs.*

What is true of America is, of course, also true of other western countries, even though they may operate a different health care system. Until the paradigm shift takes places, a large percentage of the resources currently devoted to medical care is effectively being wasted on unnecessary treatments.

In the United Kingdom, where the National Health Service is under constant pressure, just imagine the benefits if a substantial proportion of the stretched budgets could be redirected away from certain drug treatments and be released to be used in other vital areas of care.

So I invite you to share the information in this book with your relatives and friends. You will be doing them a favour. By responding positively to this invitation, you will be at the same time helping to reduce health care costs by at least 60 per cent. *It is criminal that at the end of the twentieth century, human thirst for water is still being treated with slow poisons.*

I have a request. If the information in this book helps you, please write me a note (care of the British publisher, Tagman Press) about your particular condition and how increased water intake has helped you. We need to document as much information on chronic dehydration as is possible. It is a very young science. It needs the input of all who test the information.

Your participation will save others with similar problems from the unnecessary suffering that local unidentified dehydration can produce. Like the letters printed in this book, your input can illuminate the path of others in the future.

Based on the above physiological approach to disease emergence, it is now possible to *take a resolute stand to end major dehydration-produced diseases on earth within two decades*. The public must demand the paradigm change and adopt the new paradigm to free mankind from all the 'scientific' misconceptions perpetuated for profit-motivated business expansion within the health care system. My colleagues in the medical profession must similarly stop treating the signals of dehydration of the body by the indiscriminate use of pharmaceutical products or invasive procedures.

Author's postscript

I was born in 1931 in Tehran, Iran. In 1946, only months after the Second World War, I was sent to an exclusive secondary school in Edinburgh, Scotland. Despite competition from returning servicemen, I entered St Mary's Hospital Medical School at London University as a second year student in 1951. Upon completion of my studies, I was given the privilege of being selected as one of the house doctors in my own medical school, before subsequently returning home.

The need of Iran for modern facilities was far greater than anything available within the health care system at the time, and I decided the creation of hospitals, medical and sports centres was the most important way to help in meeting the urgent health needs of the public. Immediately before the revolution of 1979, I was engaged in completion of a family charity medical centre, the largest medical complex in the country.

The revolutionary government of Iran decided to put me in prison and confiscate all personal and family assets. To do so, they levelled all types of accusations, and prepared the grounds to execute me. However, once the revolutionary guards realised that I was useful as a resident doctor among the prisoners, they delayed the execution until a later date.

I have already described in the Introduction to this book those dramatic circumstances in which I made my initial discovery about water's curative powers. Despite the difficult circumstances, for the next 25 months I became completely engrossed in clinical research of the medicinal values of water in stress reduction, and treatment of stress-related disease conditions of the body in Evin Prison, 'a most ideal stress laboratory'. The time for my trial came, and I had to answer 32 fictitious indictments carrying the death penalty. As my final defence, I presented the judge with an article on water treatment of peptic ulcer disease. To my great relief, my life was spared so that I could continue this research.

That article I wrote in prison was eventually published in the *Iranian Medical Council Journal* in 1982. A copy was also sent to

London where it was translated and then sent to the professor of gastroenterology at Yale University. The report of my discovery was later published as the guest editorial in the *Journal Of Clinical Gastroenterology* in June of 1983 and reported on in the science section of *The New York Times.*

In June of 1982, I was released from prison. Several months later, I decided to escape from Iran and go to America in order to research further and eventually introduce my medical discovery to scientists and researchers in the United States.

Nature had revealed the curative effects of simple tap water, a hitherto concealed phenomenon and in 1983, acting with the help of one supporter, I set up the Foundation for the Simple in Medicine to foster research into this topic and attempt to of change the present structure of medicine.

In 1987, after five years of constant evaluation of recent scientific literature in America, I presented a guest lecture entitled *Pain:A Need for Paradigm Change* to a select group of cancer researchers from Europe and America who had gathered in Greece. In essence, the theme of this book was presented to a body of scientists, and an article was published in the *Journal of Anticancer Research* in 1987.

In 1989, I was invited to present my discovery on pain signals of the body to scientists at the Third Interscience World Conference on Inflammation, Antirheumatics, Analgesics, and Immunomodulators. My presentation to the conference, *Neurotransmitter Histamine:An Alternative View Point*, the abstract of which was published in the conference book and distributed to thousands of research centres, explained the primary water regulatory roles of the neurotransmitter histamine. In 1989, 1990, and 1991, the Foundation's researched views on water metabolism disturbance and disease production in the body were published in an annual volume under the title of *Science in Medicine Simplified.* I had also started a campaign for public awareness of the signal systems associated with chronic dehydration.

In 1992, I was invited back to Iran and was allowed to present my views on television. I also addressed professionals at Tehran University and in teaching hospitals. Since then, my book entitled *Water Therapy* in my native language has been reprinted nine times in

Iran and the Iranian public is testing the simplicity with which water can cure many of their medical problems. Strong public reaction has forced most of the professionals to move away from their traditional use of drugs, when water by itself will do.

By writing this book, I intended to raise public awareness of the disease-producing effects of chronic dehydration on the human body. Once people become aware of the paradigm shift in medicine and begin to realise *there are no commercial aims* in encouraging them to treat the dehydration of their bodies with water, a science-based transformation of the health care system might eventually become a welcome reality.

However, one of the more obvious reasons why medicine has become so complicated and costly is the fact that the research and production of pharmaceutical products – and eventually their patient evaluation – has become monumentally expensive. To boost the sales of regularly and heavily advertised products, not only do highly paid medical representatives present their sales pitch, but doctors are also enticed into prescribing the drugs by the 'perks' offered. Patients continue to use them because they are not cured. They are not supposed to be cured! They are only treated! This is the ideal way that commercialism in medicine can thrive, and this is not the only shameful loose end.

Techniques-oriented advancements in medicine are made possible as a result of 'gadget' production. This, too, adds to the overall cost of medicine. Teaching hospitals and research institutions depend heavily on funding from the industrial side of the health-care system. Thus, research in medicine has traditionally been directed according to the wishes of health-care industrialists who release funds for their own profit-generating projects.

Now comes a moment of great rejoicing. It has been discovered that the human body possesses a variety of sophisticated indicators when it runs short of water – emergency indicators of dehydration and thirst.

The body has many more than the one 'dry mouth' indicator of water shortage. Equally obviously, the greatest tragedy in medical history is the fact that medical professionals have not understood the human body's variety of calls for water. They have traditionally resorted to chemicals and 'procedures' for dealing with chronic dehydration. A monumental mistake, but a blatant fact! The unkindest cut of all is the way in which the mainstream medical community still prefers to adhere to business as usual and ignore the good news.

Fundamentally, this basic ignorance of the manifestations of the water needs of the human body is in my opinion the primary reason for the high cost of health care in our society, without a hope of improvement in the way it is presently designed – a very bad design that only serves its operators and not the health-care-needing public.

If you look at the letters exchanged with the American Medical Association (AMA), printed in the Appendix, you will realise that well before the publication of this book, the AMA was invited to become the harbinger of the good news to the public: 'You are not sick, you are thirsty'. They remain silent.

The National Institute of Health (NIH), the most advanced centre of medical research in the world, has failed society even more miserably. Firstly, why has it not studied the medicinal effects of water? Why has it not separated the possible positive impact of water taken to swallow a pill from the medication itself? Why has it not studied what happens to a person who does not regularly drink water? These were their initial mistakes.

In May of 1989, I wrote to Dr James Mason, Assistant Secretary of Health and Human Services, explaining that a paradigm change that looked at water needs of the body would expose many solutions to the health problems of our society. I sent much supportive material, which he referred to Dr John T Kalberer, NIH Coordinator for Health Promotion and Disease Prevention, to review and discuss with me; obviously the right office for the evaluation of my revolutionary physiology-based views.

Not so! I was invited to visit with Dr Kalberer. After one hour's discussion, Dr Kalberer informed me that the NIH was not in any position to handle my 'broad' medical views.

He explained that the NIH could not fund research other than in university settings. I indicated that the reason for my contact with Dr Mason and himself was to explain dehydration as the cause of so many degenerative diseases of the human body, so that the NIH could begin its study and take the result to the public. He then told me that the NIH was only interested in the molecular aspects of biological and pharmaceutical research. He indicated my views were so broad-based they did not fit into the way the research institution functioned. When he saw I was unhappy with his pronouncement, he advised me to continue my work and publish my views. He told me this would be the only way those views would ever be heard.

I did not give up. Every time a health article appeared in newspapers based on pronouncements from someone at the NIH, I wrote and explained the basic problem. I even wrote to the Office of Scientific Integrity at the NIH and complained about some misinformation that would have established one particular product on the medical market. I did not hear from them.

For a while, I became excited when Dr Bernadine Healy became the director of the NIH. She appeared to be the right type of person who would change the NIH. As an MD and scientist, she understood what I was saying. She referred me to Stephen Croft, PhD, who had just become a temporary director of the newly established Office of Alternative Medicine until a permanent MD director could be found.

He seemed a very sincere person. After a long meeting and my having provided him with some of my published materials, he then invited me to make a presentation at the first Alternative Medicine Conference to be convened by the NIH. His temporary position was too temporary to do any good. Dr Joseph Jacobs took over. He is a doctor of medicine with Native Indian culture and influence. I am positive that Dr Croft passed my information and materials to him.

The next Alternative Medicine Conference was convened by Dr Jacobs and his second in command, and at that time I was supposed to be introduced to them by Dr Croft. Naturally, at that moment, Dr Jacobs did not have the time to conduct a serious discussion. It was agreed that he take a look at what I had sent the Office and for us to meet at a time soon.

At our meeting in his office, it became clear that he had not had the opportunity to see what I had sent. The meeting threatened to be a waste of time, but he invited me to sit down and explain my views. Before I left, he asked for another set of supportive materials, which I gave to him. Among the materials supplied was a copy of the first edition of this book. I explained to him that this information is becoming public knowledge. I invited him for the sake of society and the advancement of medical science to begin a study of the topic through his Office. I did not hear from Dr Jacobs or see him until the next Alternative Medicine Conference. Nothing about chronic dehydration was on the agenda. Even when Colonel Robert Sanders, who is very well versed with the topic, made a five-minute philosophic presentation on dehydration, no steps were taken to put the issue before the Advisory Board. It became very clear that the Office of Alternative Medicine had its own agenda and it did not appear to me that serving the public was on its list of priorities.

According to Rita Mae Brown, 'The definition of insanity is doing the same thing over and over again and expecting the results to be different.' One would assume that according to this definition, I am one of the insane ones. I often think myself to be a simpleton.

Why do I spend time and personal resources to bring about a science based transformation of medicine in, of all places, America? In the next breath I console myself by thinking I am privy to vital health and wellness information that has to reach those trusting people who become sick and do not know they are only thirsty for water. With this thought I go the next stretch of my weary way.

In the meantime, Dr Bernadine Healy left the NIH. She is a medical doctor. The NIH is a 'science' institution. Obviously there must have been a conflict of purpose. Nobel Laureate Harold Varmus took over. In November 1993, I wrote to him. I started my letter: 'Welcome to the position that you can now make a greater contribution to advancement of medical science and our society. Today's *Washington Post* article on you prompted me to write this letter and bring a breakthrough of significance in medical science to your attention. "It is chronic dehydration that is the root cause of most major diseases." I have in the past tried to get the NIH to take a serious look at this simple "paradigm shift" and make the future practice of medicine patient-friendly!' I sent him one of my books and supportive materials, but received no reply – not even an acknowledgement.

The only way to take the 'dehydration message' to the public was by writing. That I did. After sending letters to various journals and newspapers and not hearing from them, I decided in 1989 to create a journal at the Foundation for the Simple in Medicine. We called it *Science in Medicine Simplified*. A special issue and a regular issue were published in a period of one year and freely distributed to some research centres and medical libraries at universities.

We also applied to the National Library of Medicine for the journals to be indexed in the Index Medicus computer system, so that their content could be accessed by other researchers. We appealed to them to afford us an equal opportunity to present our 'paradigm shift' researched views in medicine. They got back to us and said two volumes of a publication were not enough, but once another volume was put out and we were sure there was going to be continuity they would consider indexing the journals.

The third volume of the journal was in preparation and, when it was published in 1991, we sent our application and two volumes of each publication to the NLM. Journals are evaluated two to three times a year for their possible inclusion in the Index Medicus. The committee consists of mainly NIH scientists. When they met at the end of the year and reviewed our new information in medicine, we were refused. They did not want to give us an equal opportunity for our views to be heard. The NIH 'thinkers' did not wish our new thoughts to enter the scientific arena and eventually reach the public. We were deftly censored. This is when I decided to write the first edition of this book and 'go public'.

About six months after the NLM refusal, my book was out and being reviewed. I now had a simple language explanation of where mainstream medicine had gone wrong. This was the book I sent, in addition to the scientific publications, to Drs Healy, Croft and Jacobs at the NIH. I wanted them to know I did not need them for my views to reach the public.

In April 1993, there was an International Bio-Oxidative Medical Conference in Reston, Virginia. This is a conference convened by practitioners of alternative medicine, and I was invited to speak following the President of the Association. I was introduced to one of the NIH Scientific Secretaries, Dr Edmund Sargent Copeland, who had been invited to review the conference. After my talk on the role of histamine as the body's main water regulator, he graciously discussed how I could succeed in getting my views evaluated. I sent him most of my published materials. We met at their Westbard Avenue office. He did his best to get me invited by the programme manager of their lectures to speak before their members. The invitation never came.

I have tried to give you detailed information about my efforts to get the people who are entrusted with the responsibility of looking after America's health interests to work on behalf of the public, and I hope that readers of this book will become a part of the force behind the transformation of America's health care system.

Obviously, funding for the evaluation of water as a natural medicine seems not to be readily available. Furthermore, even if funds were to be made available, research of the topic seems not attractive enough to the universities and nationally recognised research centres. And yet, to show others, patient response to treatment with water as a natural medicine in diseases produced by chronic dehydration is necessary. It is necessary to convince the clinicians within the health care system to change their present approach to treatment. Students in medical schools are still not taught anything about the many roles of water in the human body.

The way I see it, we need many 'simple and direct' observations, like those from people whose letters are published in this book, before mainstream medical practitioners would even consider abandoning their method of treatment. Their present method is only suited to promotion of chemical products. 'Double-blind randomised trials' are only suited to the evaluation of one chemical product to another, less known substance. This particular methodology is not suited to the clinical evaluation of 'deficiency disorders', in this case the effects of water on the variety of dehydration-produced diseases.

The physiological state of each individual's body determines the initial symptoms and complications of dehydration. That is why these symptom-producing dehydration states have traditionally been labelled as many different disease conditions.

But new research that was published in February 2000 has

revealed an important relationship between water/salt consumption and sustained activation of the sympathetic nervous system and the body's adrenalin production. When water by itself activates the production of adrenalin, it directs the body toward physical activity and tissue reconstruction, a most positive effect. It reverses the impact of dehydration and its associated tissue breakdown that is fundamental to eventual disease production in the body. By sustained activation of the adrenergic nerve system, water acts as a natural inhibitor of histamine's over-activity that is reponsible for manifesting its drought management programmes of the body – labelled 'diseases' such as asthma, allergies, lupus, adult onset diabetes and other auto-immune diseases.

When it activates the body's adrenergic system within five minutes of its adequate intake, water exposes its superior emergency medicinal value in severe asthma attacks. The patient should no longer need to visit the hospital casualty department to receive an intravenous saline solution and an injection of adrenalin to abort the attack. Concurrently, when the adrenergic system is activated and adrenalin secretion ensues, certain enzyme systems that regulate the body's metabolism are also stimulated into activity. One of these enzyme systems involves the activation of a fat-breaking-and-burning enzyme called hormone sensitive lipase. When present in the blood, this acts on cholesterol plaques and causes them to shrink and eventually disappear. Thus, water by itself is the best anti-cholesterol medication.

It seems that when water by itself enters the body, it can raise blood pressure. However, if salt is made available to the body, the rise is not significant. This research finding supports my view that salt is essential for the body and has 'blood pressure lowering effect' – a view contrary to presently held medical opinion.

The letters in this book on water's role in the cure of asthma and allergies, weight loss, cholesterol reduction and anginal pain are proof of the above-mentioned actions of adequate water intake, among many others. I continue to receive many letters, and value them all for the support they offer and the personal evidence they contribute. As I write, there is an e-mail on my desk from a Hindu Monastery in Hawaii that begins 'Aloha Dr Batmanghelidj'. It seems that my water treatment method is in total harmony with the traditional Hindu system of medicine called Ayurveda. Yet the head of the monastery admitted that they had not been aware that tea and coffee did not hydrate the body adequately. Since adopting the practice of drinking adequate plain water daily, the health, digestion, alterness, sleep and even meditations of all the monks had improved. Furthermore, the Abbot wants to recommend my book to the worldwide Hindu congregation. I also receive letters regularly from British readers and one writer asked recently why the National Health Service in the UK did not adopt these same methods as they seem to offer massive savings in government health expenditure.

One further comment regarding the chapter on AIDS. Despite all the recent research the problem still remains, in my opinion, a metabolic disorder. I feel my research is as valid today as it was 14 years ago. As you have seen in Figure 16 (page 124), protease enzymes are involved in the breakdown of tissues. They are activated by sustained secretion of cortisone-activating neurotransmitters that eventually cause depletion of some body reserves. Unfortunately, the current approach to AIDS treatment mandates the intake of protease inhibitors, but does not encourage the physiologic/metabolic reversal of the process that causes continued protease activation and drastic tissue breakdown.

In conclusion, I should like to repeat that we are now at the dawn of a new era in medical science. It is chronic water shortage in the body that causes most of the diseases of the human body. The original design of the human body is more complete than you can imagine. If we have not known how to maintain it until now, it is our own fault. We have not stopped to think – if the body is mainly water, where will it get its top-up if we don't drink water on a regular basis? We now know when it is calling for urgent water intake. We need to dwell on this information There is no hidden agenda to the promotion of this vital message. If you choose to share this information with loved ones, you will be its beneficiaries.

At present this book is the only source of easy-to-read-and-understand information on chronic dehydration. You need to read it a few times to understand the profound nature of the indispensable role of water in the human body.

If you do this, you will become a healer too. If you have found the information in this book useful, please raise your voice. Doctors are supposed to be healers. They have taken an oath to serve mankind. It is true that the 'business of America is business', but my business-minded colleagues have no right to obstruct my simple message that: 'You are not sick, you are thirsty' from reaching a wider public.

I humbly acknowledge that not all doctors put their own gain before the welfare of those who seek their honest advice. But a very small minority, unfortunately in steering positions, have shed a bad light on our profession. However, 'when light comes, darkness has to go'.

Traditionally, doctors have been thinkers and philosophers. It is only recently that they have been forced to memorise pre-digested information to get through the curriculum in teaching hospitals. In reality, books are created to store information, and the brain is designed to think. Once we get rid of the burden of having to remember so much misinformation generated around the conditions that are complications of chronic dehydration, doctors will once again become scholars and thinkers.

In the hope of a new era of bright lights in medicine, I wish the readers of this book luck in their efforts to assist the transformation of the present structure of medicine. Each letter that is published in the book is but a sample of what 'water as medicine' can do for millions who present similar outward manifestations of chronic dehydration. The arrogant and the ignorant in medical practice will label these letters as 'anecdotal' and brush them aside. Infinitely greater in number, seeing eyes connected to thinking brains will recognise in each one of them the new truth: 'You are not sick, you are thirsty'.

This book, I should say finally, is is not designed to be read for soundbites. That is the reason why it does not have an index. It should be read ideally as a love story, like a novel, which describes in detail the beautiful and compelling love relationship between water and the human body.

F Batmanghelidj, MD
Falls Church, Virginia
March 2000

Appendix

In 1990, the president and board members of the American Medical Association were sent an invitation by the Foundation for the Simple in Medicine to share information provided on the paradigm shift on water metabolism of the body with their active medical colleagues. This letter of invitation was subsequently published in the 1991 issue of *Science in Medicine Simplified*. It is also presented below with subsequent correspondences with AMA. You are now being informed of some of the actions taken to bring my findings about chronic dehydration to the public through the members of the AMA.

This is an invitation you should forcefully extend to your doctor and administrators of health-care systems. More than enough scientific information to demand necessary change in the present structure of the health care system is now available. Please do not be indifferent to the pain and suffering of others. Take a resolute stand.

C John Tupper, MD
President
American Medical Association
24 July 1990

Dear Dr Tupper:
The present status of clinical medicine seems to draw much criticism from the health-care needing but dissatisfied public; and the tax payers who have to endure the spiraling health-care costs. Kathryn Welling's June 11 article in BARRON'S further reflects the problem into the dismal future. The situation does not need to be so abysmally hopeless. All it takes to restructure the seemingly hopeless situation to abundantly hopeful and full of science blessed possibilities is a simple paradigm change in the basic understanding of the physiology of the human body, and its application to the practice of clinical medicine. The highlights of the paradigm change are the following.
The human body has a major problem with its normal water

regulation, caused by a gradual loss of thirst sensation. This problem is confronted often enough in clinical practice that it does not need explanation. However, The Lancet *Editorial of 3 November 1984 and the 20 September 1984 article by Paddy Phillips are enclosed to remove any doubt on the issue. If water is important to the human body, then its loss must leave some hall marks that need clarification. With the existence of such water deprived states, without full attention to the complex primary water intake and distribution systems of the body, to chemically tamper with the individual water regulators within the same systems would not be in the best interest of the persons who are being clinically treated, more so when these systems become so openly signal producing!*

The published abstract of my presentation on the neurotransmitter histamine and the content of the publication Science in Medicine Simplified *attempt at covering some of the proposed pertinent details on the above discussion. As a sympathetic colleague, I invite you to take a very serious look at the already exposed paradigm change. Also, from the position of leadership and trust that your active professional colleagues have bestowed on you, invite them to study the paradigm change and apply it to patient care. My clinical and theoretical studies expose that a paradigm shift – from a total scientific attention directed at the particulate solutes in the body, to the study of the different systems' disturbance caused by its signal producing solvent metabolism malregulation – will pave the way for the development of very many effective solutions to major health-care problems of the society.*

The presently held paradigm, that permits a physician to maltreat the signals of simple body water deficiency and its projections of need with cocktails of pharmaceutical products, is inadequate for dealing with the needs and the problems of the chronically dehydrated sick. It is not prestige enhancing for the clinicians either. Moreover, it is to the absurd disadvantage of the society in which we all try to live without the fear of becoming tax-broken, because of the compounding results of an inherited elementary mistake in the science of physiology. The time to act and shed bias is now, if an orderly paradigm shift is professionally desirable!

Time consuming silence, hesitation, complacency, or even emotional rejection of the paradigm shift by the professionals in clinical practice, and policy making positions, will only invite poignant public criticism in the near future.

I hope my serious enthusiasm at initially inviting colleagues to adopt the paradigm shift is reflective of sincere professional good will. It is appreciated that an orderly change is very desirable. However, on the basis of its generated scientific information, this Foundation does not consider the continuance of the status quo in the practice of clinical medicine to the best interest of the society. We therefore invite you to begin the establishment of a program for the evaluation and adoption of our exposed paradigm change by the members of the American Medical Association.

With very best wishes for your success in the realisation of new possibilities through a science based paradigm shift approach to the health care needs of the society. Your comments would clear the next step of the way and direction for the public needed establishment of the new paradigm.

Sincerely,

F Batmanghelidj
Foundation for the Simple in Medicine

Copy:
Other AMA Officers and Members of the Board of Trustees
Senator Pryor, Special Committee On Aging
Dr Louis Sullivan
Public Awareness Committee of the Foundation

Enclosures:
BARRON'S 11 June Editorial Article by Kathryn M Welling
Lancet *Editorial, 3 November 1984*
Article by Paddy A Phillips, et. al.
New England Journal of Medicine, 20 September 1984
Abstract, Neurotransmitter Histamine:An Alternative View Point
Science in Medicine Simplified, Volume 1, April 1990

Following is the text of the reply from Dr C John Tupper, MD, President of the AMA.

AMA
August 28, 1990
F Batmanghelidj, MD
Foundation for the Simple in Medicine

Dear Dr Batmanghelidj:
This is in reply to your letter of July 24 in which you present your concepts on water regulation and the problems associated with body water deficiency, particularly in the elderly. I will share this information with members of our staff.
Thank you for keeping us informed of your activities.
Sincerely,
C John Tupper, MD

I did not think the above letter showed sincerity to the cause of advancement in medicine. I decided to publish my letter to Dr Tupper and his response in the Journal of the Foundation and send a copy of the Journal with the following letter to Dr John Ring, then elected AMA president.

John J Ring, MD
President
American Medical Association
21 August 1991

Dear Dr Ring:
I have pleasure in sending you a copy of the 1991 issue of Science in Medicine Simplified (SMS). *In 1990, we invited the American Medical Association to begin an evaluation of our exposed paradigm shift in human applied research. We found the response of Dr Tupper, then President of AMA, non committal, evasive and lacking in substance. We decided to publish the text of the letter of invitation and its response in the 1991 issue of SMS. It is now a*

recorded fact that through a paradigm change, we introduced a science-based solution to some of the health problems of the society to AMA, a qualified body of people whose business it is to find simpler ways of curing disease. From here on, it is up to you to justify the reasons why AMA failed to investigate and bring out the possible simpler solutions to health problems that the evaluation of the paradigm change could offer the public - the public that is in a desperate need of a better and cheaper health care system, and we in the medical profession have taken an oath to give it to them.
Sincerely,
F Batmanghelidj

I received the following response from Dr Roy Schwarz of the AMA.

M Roy Schwarz, MD, Senior Vice President,
Medical Education & Science
September 11, 1991

F Batmanghelidj, MD
Foundation for the Simple in Medicine

Dear Doctor Batmanghelidj:
Thank you so much for your letter of August 21, 1991 that was addressed to John J. Ring, MD. I will pass the journal that you enclosed, 'Science in Medicine Simplified', to appropriate science staff for information here at the American Medical Association (AMA). The AMA appreciates being informed of your efforts.
Sincerely,
M. Schwarz, MD

Needless to say, nothing has been done to prevent the use of chemicals for the treatment of chronic dehydration in the human body. Unless people begin to show their strong objections to the continuation of this 'sting', society will continue to suffer from ill health and a great deal of wasted health-care expenditure.

Bibliography

References from: F Batmanghelidj: *Is Cell Membrane Receptor Protein Down-Regulation Also a Hydrodynamic Phenomenon?*, *Science In Medicine Simplified*, Vol. 2, June 1991 are selected as the main bibliography for this book. This article attempts to present aspects of the long-term damage of an established and expanding dehydration in the human body. The content of this book reflects on these and several hundred other articles. These articles can be used more coherently and fit a pattern, in the light of the paradigm shift which has a background of extensive clinical observations.

Batmanghelidj F; *Pain: A Need for Paradigm Change*; *Anticancer Research*, Vol. 7, No. 5B, pages 971–990, September/October1987.

Editorial; *Thirst And Osmoregulation in the Elderly*, pages 1017-1018, *Lancet*, November 1984.

Steen B, Lundgren B K, Isaksson B; *Body Water In The Elderly*; page 101, *Lancet*, January 12, 1985.

Phillips P A, Rolls B J, Ledingham J G G, Forsling M L, Morton J J, Crowe M J and Wollner L; *Reduced Thirst After Water Deprivation in the Elderly Men*; *The New England Journal Of Medicine*, pages 753–759, Vol. 311, No. 12, September 20, 1984.

Bruce A, Anderson M, Arvidsson B and Isaksson B; *Body Composition. Prediction of Normal Body Potassium, Body Water and Body Fat In Adults on the Basis of Body Height, Body Weight and Age*; *Scand. J. Clin. Lab. Invest.* 40, pages 461–473, 1980.

Humes H D; *Disorders Of Water Metabolism; Fluids' and Electrolytes*, Eds Kokko and Tannen, Saunders, pages 118-149, 1986.
Katchalski-Katzir E; *Conformational Change In Macromolecules*; *Biorheology*, 21, pages 57-74, 1984.

Srivastava D K and Bernhard S A; *Enzyme-Enzyme Interaction And The Regulation Of Metabolic Reaction Pathways*; Current topics In Cellular Regulation, Vol. 28, pages 1–68, 1986.

Rimon G, Hanski E, Braun S, and Levitzki A; *Mode of Coupling between Hormone Receptors and Adenylate Cyclase Elucidated by Modulation of Membrane Fluidity*; Nature, Vol. 276, pages 396–396, 23 November, 1978.

Hanski E, Rimon G and Levitzki A; *Adenylate Cyclase Activation by the Beta-Adrenergic Receptors as a Diffusion-Controlled Process*; American Chemical Society, Vol. 18, No. 5, pages 846–853, 1979.
Ross E M and Gilman A G; *Biochemical Properties of Hormone-Sensitive Adenylate Cyclase*; Ann. Rev. Biochem., 49, pages 533–564, 1980.

Wiggins P M; *A Mechanism of ATP-Driven Cation Pumps*; pages 266-269, *Biophysics of Water*, Eds Felix Franks and Sheila F Mathis, John Wiley And Sons Ltd, 1982.

Tada M, Masa-Aki Kadoma, Makoto Inui, Makoto Yamada and Fumio Ohmori; *Ca2+ dependent ATPase of the Sarcoplasmic Reticulum*; pages 137-164, *Transport and Bio-energetics in Biomembranes*, Eds Ray Sato & Yasuo Kagawa, Plenum Press N.Y., London, 1982.

Yellen G; *Permeation in Potassium Channels: Implications For Channel Structure*; Annu. Rev. Biophys. Biophys Chem., 16, pages 227–46, 1987.

Finkelstein A; *Water Movement Through Lipid Bilayers, Pores and Plasma Membrane, Theory and Reality*; Distinguished Lecture Series of the Society of General Physiologists, Vol. 4, John Wiley & Sons Ltd, 1987.

Stryer L; *Introduction to Biological Membranes*, pages 205-253, *Biochemistry*, W H Freedman and Company, 1981.

Rand R P, and Parsegian V A; *Phospholipid Bilayer Hydration - Interbilayer Repulsion and Interbilayer Structural Changes*, pages 140-143, *Biophysics Of Water,* Eds Felix Franks and Sheila F Mathis, John Wiley & Sons Ltd, 1982.

Silver B L; *The Physical Chemistry of Membranes,* The Solomon Press, NY and Allen & Unwin, (Boston, London, Sydney).

Sek-Wen Hui; *Ultrastructural Studies of The Molecular Assembly in Biomembranes: Diversity and Similarity, Current Topics In Membranes & Transport,* Vol. 29, pages 29-70, Academic Press, 1987. Edidin M; *Rotational & Lateral Diffusion of Membrane Proteins and Lipids: Phenomena and Function*; pages 91-127, *Current Topics in Membranes & Transport,* Vol. 29, pages 29-70, Academic Press, 1987.

Rolf-C Gaillard and Saad Al-Damluji; *Stress And The Pituitary-Adrenal Axis*, pages 319-354, *Ballier's Clinical Endocrinology and Metabolism,* Vol.1 No.2, May 1987.

Eisenman G; *An Introduction to Molecular Architecture and Permeability of Ion Channels*; pages 205-26, *Ann. Rev. Biophys. Biophys. Chem.* 16, 1987.

Sowers A E and Hackenbrock C R; *Rate of Lateral Diffusion of Intramembrane Particles: Measurement by Electrophoretic Displacement and Rerandomization*; *Proc. Natl. Acad. Sci. USA.,* Vol. 78, No. 10, pages 6246-6250, cell biology, 1981.

Garner J A and Mahler H R; *Biogenesis of Presynaptic Terminal Proteins*; *Journal of Neurochemistry;* 49, pages 905-915, 1987.

Weiss D G and Gross G W; *Intracellular Transport In Nerve Process: The Chromatographic Dynamics Of Axoplasmic Transport*; pages 387-396, *Biological Structure and Coupled Flows,* Eds A Oplaka and M Balaban, Academic Press, 1983.

Vale R D, Reese T S and Sheetz M P; *Identification of a Novel Force-Generating Protein, Kinesin, involved in Microtubule-based Motility*; *Cell* Vol. 42, pages 39-50, 1985.

Porter M E, Scholey J M, Stemple D L, Vigers G-PA, Vale R D et al; *Characterization of the Microtubule Movement produced by Sea Urchin Egg Kinesin*; *The Journal of Biological Chemistry*, Vol. 262, No. 6, pages 2794-2802, February 25, 1987.

Gross G W and Weiss G; *Theoretical Considerations on Rapid Transport in Low Viscosity Axonal Regions*; pages 330-341, *Axoplasmic Transport*, Ed D G Weiss, Spriger-Verlag 1982.

Weiss D G; *The Mechanism of Axoplasmic Transport* (Chapter 20), pages 275-307, *Axoplasmic Transport*, Ed Zafar Iqbal, PhD, CRC Press Inc, 1987.

Ochs S; *On The Mechanism of Axoplasmic Transport*, pages 342-349, *Axoplasmic Transport*, Ed D G Weiss, Spriger-Verlag 1982.

Sauve R, Simoneau C, Parent L, Monette R and Roy G; *Oscillatory Activation of Calcium-Dependent Channels In HeLa Cells Induced by Histamine H1 Receptor Stimulation: A Single Channel Study*; *J. Membrane Biol.*, 96, 199-208, 1987.

Laczi F, Ivanyi T, Julesz J, Janaky T and Laszlo F A; *Plasma Arginin-8-Vasopressin Response to Osmotic or Histamine Stimulation Contribute to the Differential Diagnosis of Central Diabetes Insipidus*; *Acta Endocrinologica* (Copenh), 113, pages 168-174, 1986.

Espiner E A; *The Effect of Stress on Salt and Water Balance*; pages 375-390, *Ballier's Clinical Endocrinology and Metabolism*, Vol.1 No.2, May 1987.

Mellgren R; *Calcium-Dependent Proteases: An Enzyme System Active At Cellular Membranes?*; *FASEB J.* 1, pages110-115; 1987.

Rega A F; *Transport of Ca2+ and ATP Hydrolysis by the Calcium Pump*; pages 67-90, *The Ca2+ Pump of Plasma Membranes;* Eds Alcides F Rega And Patricio J Garrahan, CRC Press 1986.

Van Rossum G D V, Russo M A and Schisselbauer J C; *Role of Cytoplasmic Vesicles in Volume Maintenance*; Current Topics In Membranes & Transport, Vol. 30, pages 45-74,Academic Press, 1987.

Mellman I, Howe C and Helenius A; *The Control of Membrane Traffic on the Endocytic Pathway*; Current Topics In Membranes and Transport. Vol. 29, pages 255-288,Academic Press, 1987.

Lefkowitz R J, and Caron M G; *Regulation of Adrenergic Receptor Function by Phosphorylation*; Current Topics In Cellular Regulation, Vol. 28, pages 209-231,Academic Press, 1986.

Mizumoto T; *Effects of the Calcium Ion on the Wound Healing Process*; Current Topics in Hokkaido Igaku Zasshi, 62,Vol.2, pages 332-45, March 1987.

Kahlson G,Rosengren E & WhiteT; *The Formation of Histamine in the Rat Foetus;J. Physiol,* Vol. 151, pages 131-138, 1960.

Kahlson G, Rosengren E and Steinhardt C; *Histamine-Forming Capacity of Multiplying Cells*; J. Physiol, Vol.169, pages 487-498,1963.

Haartmann U V, Kahlson G & Stinhardt C; *Histamine Formation In Germinating Seeds*; Life Sciences, Vol. 5, pages 1-9, 1966.

Kahlson G and Rosengren E; *Histamine Formation as related to Growth and Protein*; Biogenic Amines As Physiological Regulators; Ed J J Blum, 223-238, 1970.

Brandes L J, Bogdanovic R P, Cawker M D and Labella F S; *Histamine and Growth: Interaction of Antiestrogen Binding Site Ligands with* a Novel Histamine Site that may be associated with Calcium Channels; Cancer Research, Vol. 47, pages 4025-4031, August 1987.

Goldstein D J, Marante Perez D J, Gunst J P and Halperin J A; Increase In Mast Cell Number and Altered Vascular Permeability in Thirsty Rats; Life Sciences, Vol. 23, pages 1591-1602, August 1978.

Izumi H, Ho S-H, Michelakis A M and Aoki T; Different Effects of Compound 48/80 and Histamine on Plasma Renin Activity; European Journal of Pharmacology, 91, 295-299, 1983.

Zaloga G P, Chernow B and Eil C; Hypercalcemia and Disseminated Cytomegalovirus Infection in the Acquired Immunedeficiency Syndrome; Annals Of Internal Medicine, 102, pages 331-333, 1985.

Jacob M B; The Acquired Immunedeficiency Syndrome and Hypercalcemia, West J. Med., 144, pages 469-471, April 1986.

Biochemical Pathways Index, Boehringer, Manheim.

Watterson J G: The Role of Water in Cell Architecture, Molecular and Cellular Biochem. 79: 101-105, 1988.

Iqbal M J; Regulatory Role of Cellular Free Water; Science In Medicine Simplified, Vol. 1, PP. 41-54, A Foundation for the Simple in Medicine Publication, April 1990.

Batmanghelidj F; Neurotransmitter Histamine: An Alternative View Point; Science In Medicine Simplified, a Foundation for the Simple in Medicine Publication, Vol. 1, pages 8-39, April 1990.

Robertson R P and Chen M A; Role for Prostaglandin E in Defective Insulin Secretion and Carbohydrate Intolerance in Diabetes Mellitus; J. Clin. Invest., 60, pages 747-753, 1973.

Robertson R P, Tsai P, Little S A, Zhang H J and Walseth T F; Receptor-

Mediated Adenylate Cyclase-Coupled Mechanism for PGE2 Inhibition of Insulin Secretion in HIT Cells; Diabetes, Vol. 36, pages 1047-1053, 1987.

Robertson R P; *Eicosanoids as Pluripotential Modulators of Pancreatic Islet Function; Diabetes,* Vol. 37, pages 367-370, 1988.
Weir G C and Bonner-Weir S; *Islets of Langerhans: The Puzzle of Intraislet Interactions and their Relevance to Diabetes; J. Clin. Invest.* Volume 85, pages 983-987, April 1990.

Iqbal M J; *Tryptophan; Science In Medicine Simplified,* Vol. 1, pages 55-78, a Foundation for the Simple in Medicine Publication, April 1990.

Goodwin S J; *Prostaglandins and Host Defense in Cancer, Medical Clinics of North America,* Vol. 65, No. 4, pages 829-844, 1981.

Kavelaars A, Berkenbosch F, Croiset G, Ballieux R E and Heijnen C J; *Induction of b-Endorphin Secretion by Lymphocytes after Subcutaneous Administration of Corticotropin-Releasing Factor; Endocrinology* 126, No. 2, 759-764, 1990.

Suda T, Tozawa F, Ushiyama T, Sumitomo T, Yamada M and Demura H; *Interleukin-1 Stimulates Corticotropin-Releasing Factor Gene Expression in Rat Hypothalamus; Endocrinology* 126, No. 2, 1223-1228, 1990.

Sandler S, Bendtzen K, Eizirik D L and Welsh M; *Interleukin-6 Affects Insulin Secretion and Glucose Metabolism of Rat Pancreatic Islets in Vitro; Endocrinology* 126, No. 2, 1288-1294, 1990.

Rieckmann P, D'Alessandro F, Nordan R P, Fauci A S and Kehrl J H; *IL-6 and Tumor Necrosis Factor-a; The Journal of Immunology,* 146, 3462-68, 1991.

Hasselgren P-O, Pedersen P, Sax H C, Warner B W and Fischer J E;

Current Concepts of Protein Turnover and Amino Acid Transport in Liver and Skeletal Muscles During Sepsis; Arch Surg, 123, 992-999, 1988.

Brown J M, Grosso M A and Harken A H; *Cytokines, Sepsis and the Surgeon*; Surgery, Gynaecology & Obstetrics, 169, 568-575, December 1989.

Hempling H G; *Osmosis: The Push and Pull of Life*; pages 205-214, *Biophysics Of Water*, Eds Felix Franks and Sheila F Mathis, John Wiley & Sons Ltd, 1982.

Cicoria A D and Hempling H G; *Osmotic Properties of a Proliferating and Differentiating Line of Cells From Bone Marrow of the Rat; Membrane Permeability to Non-electrolytes*; J. Cellular Physiology 105, 105-127, 1980.

Cicoria A D and Hempling H G; *Osmotic Properties of Differentiating Bone Marrow Precursor Cells: Membrane Permeability to Non-Electrolytes*; J. Cellular Physiology 105, 120-136, 1980.

Batmanghelidj F; *A New and Natural Method of Treatment of Peptic Ulcer Disease*; J Clin Gastroentrol, 5, 203-205, 1983.

Additional information

Further copies of this book and other important books and tapes
by Dr. Batmanghelidj and other Tagman authors
may be ordered from Tagman Distribution Direct at
Lovemore House, PO Box 754, Norwich, UK NR1 4GY.
Credit Card hotlines : **01206 734372 & 01603 431432** (24 hours).
e mail **handprints@cwcom.net**
Website addresses :
www.tagman-press.com *or* **www.watercure.com**

How to Deal With Back Pain and Rheumatoid Joint Pain
Paperback book. 112 pages, 33 illustrations. £10.00.

This educational, preventive-treatment manual gives you easy-to-use techniques for relieving chronic back pain and rheumatoid joint pain. It's the ideal accompaniment to Dr. Batmanghelidj's video, *How To Deal With Back Pain*, since it illustrates and explains the easy-to-do corrective body movements for instant and lasting back pain relief.   You will learn the importance of maintaining the proper alkalinity in your body's cells and how water and salt can be used to wash away the acidity that causes pain.   You will understand the structure of your body's spinal column, vertebrae and joints - made easy with the book's clear pictures, graphics and model demonstrations. You will learn some simple, everyday techniques for preventing strained muscles and overextended ligaments, ways to strengthen back muscles and the important role of the foot and its arches in supporting the body in motion.

ABC of Asthma, Allergies and Lupus
Paperback book. 229 pages. £10.00.
This book explains the direct relationship between water deficiency in the body and asthma, allergies and lupus.

Pain: Arthritis Pain & Back Pain
Special 12 page report. £7.00.
This special report on pain explains the importance of pain as a thirst signal of the body, and why arthritis and back pain are the same dehydration-produced signals that signify a disease producing level of local drought in different regions of the body.

Asthma: Cause & Cure
Special 28 page report. £7.00.
This special report on asthma explains the new discovery that asthma is one of the major indicators of 'drought' in the body.   It describes how lack of sufficient water in the body causes constriction of the bronchioles in the lungs and how water and salt serve as its ideal medications. This special report teaches you how you can abort an asthma attack, and how water and salt have life-saving applications for asthmatics.

How to Deal With Back Pain
Video (25 minutes). £20.00.
Back pain is a common complaint that afflicts almost everyone at some time or another. This easy-to-follow programme shows you how to promote better fluid circulation in your spinal discs to gain instant relief from back pain and sciatic pain. It also outlines the latest scientific breakthroughs on the physiology of chronic back pain. The video provides step-by-step instructions to help you identify the source and location of your pain. It shows simple body exercises that actually normalise the position of the vertebral discs and draw the pain-causing disc away from the spinal cord - which will normally relieve sciatic pain within a half hour. The exercises also strengthen the 'stays of your spine', back muscles, tendons and ligaments, thus hopefully preventing further suffering.

Cure Pain and Prevent Cancer
Video (2 hours). Thomas Jefferson University Medical School. £27.00.
In this videotaped presentation at the Yoga Research Society's 1997 Conference, Dr. Batmanghelidj explains the link between chronic pain and cancer, and shows you how to use water and salt to relieve pain and prevent disease. In this enlightening presentation, he explains how pain is a cry from your body for more water and salt - and a warning sign that you could be at risk of cancer or other serious illness. New research on how your immune system becomes prone to uncontrolled cell overgrowth, DNA damage and DNA repair dysfunction that leads to cancer shows a vital dependence of your body not just on water but on salt as well. In fact, a whole host of degenerative diseases are linked not only to dehydration but also to inadequate salt intake. Dr. Batmanghelidj demonstrates exactly how much salt should be taken with water. Learn how to use water and salt in the proper balance. Learn why *pain is a thirst signal you can't afford to ignore!* Find out exactly what steps you should take to shield yourself and those close to you from pain and disease.

Water & Salt: The Miracle Medications
Video (2 hours). £27.00.
This is Dr. Batmanghelidj's intriguing presentation to the Circle of Light Foundation in 1997. Now you can learn how to replenish the oceans inside your cells with water and maintain the proper volume of water outside your cells with salt. Learn to use water and salt effectively to prevent cancer and to treat and cure arthritis, diabetes, hypertension, asthma and possibly Alzheimer's disease - and other degenerative diseases associated with aging. Understand how water and salt work together to regulate all your body's critical functions. Recognise the three stages of dehydration and how you can quickly and easily reverse the damage. Learn why both water and salt are essential together to fully prevent dangerous effects of dehydration. Discover the vital link between water and the health of your brain - learn how to put an end to foggy thinking, and reverse memory loss. Learn how drinking more water can cause excess weight to drop off, while you actually eat more of the foods you love. Feel full while your body's metabolism burns off more pounds.

Water: Rx for a Healthier, Pain-Free Life
Audio tape course and 50 page Handbook. £45.00.
This comprehensive, ten hour audiotape seminar gives you a firm foundation for Dr. Batmanghelidj's natural water cure programme. You'll get answers to the most frequently asked 'whys' and 'hows' of the water cure, and learn how it can be used to treat a surprisingly broad range of ailments. 'Dr. B.' explains in detail the body's newly discovered thirst perceptions and crisis signals of dehydration, and why so many 'disease conditions' are actually states of dehydration that can be prevented and cured by balancing one's daily water

and salt intake. These eight informative audiotapes are ideal for any-time listening - at home, on the road, or for group discussions. They are an excellent source of information for the visually impaired. The 50 page handbook serves a a guideline to the information covered in the audiotaped presentations. For best results this handbook should be read before you listen to the tapes. It will prepare your mind so you gain maximum benefit from the information presented in the seminar. This guide also serves as an invaluable reference manual to recognising your body's thirst signals .... the common health problems that often result from unintentional dehydration .... and how to treat them with the proper timing and correct proportions of water and salt.

Your Body's Many Cries For Water
Audio tape. £7.00
Dr. Batmanghelidj's lecture at the 39th PA Annual Natural Living Conference held at Kutztown University, PA, in 1993 - a lecture that received a standing ovation. Learn where and when the water cure was discovered. Learn more about Alexander Fleming's discovery of penicillin, and what he told Dr. Batmanghelidj when he was Sir Alexander's student. Learn why water can permanently erase pain and counteract the effects of stress. Discover pain-relieving properties of water and why pain is a sign of serious, system-wide dehydration. Learn how you can shut off pain without side-effect ridden drugs. You'll be inspired by the real-life examples of people who have used the 'water cure' to put an end to their pain and suffering.

Water: The New Immune Breakthrough & Pain and Cancer 'Wonder Drug'
Audio tape. £7.00
The Capital University of Integrative Medicine Postgraduate Guest Lecture. Hear what a group of postgraduate health-care professionals that included medical doctors and chiropractors, learned from 'Dr. B.' about dehydration as the primary cause of the painful degenerative diseases of the human body. Contains information on how cancer occurs when there is long-term shortage of water in the body. Includes two case histories of breast cancer and lymphoma that have gone into remission because of the patients' increased water intake.

Multiple Sclerosis: Is Water Its Cure?
Audio tape. £7.00.
Hear real-life evidence of the link between dehydration and MS. In this lively audio tape of the *Just Common Sense* radio programme hosted by Bob Butts, you will hear from a young male MS sufferer who used Dr. Batmanghelidj's water and salt programme to put an end to his symptoms. This revealing interview explains how you can use the same water and salt cure to bring relief to the incapacitating fatigue, swelling, and the vision and cognitive problems that plague MS sufferers. He also discusses the destructive effects of caffeine on memory and energy.

Readers seeking further insight into Dr. Batmanghelidj's work may like to visit his web site at **www.watercure.com**

THE TAGMAN PRESS
Books to Inspire, Excite and Transform!

The Tagman Press is a new global publishing imprint and internet book-seller founded by international bestselling author Anthony Grey. In a short time it has established a list of outstanding and controversial books that challenge conventional thinking and shed new light on vital current issues. In addition to this ground-breaking and increasingly influential book by Dr. Fereydoon Batmanghelidj, **The Tagman Press** also publishes the following titles which outline extraordinary new insights in the realms of science and spirituality.

Yes to Human Cloning *by Claude Rael*
P'back ISBN 1-903571-05-7 £10.00. Hardback ISBN 1-903571-04-9 £17.50
The author is the founder of Clonaid, the first organisation to embark on the cloning of a human being. In this extraordinary new book he describes how science is about to revolutionise all our lives in the next two decades - and asserts that cloning technology will soon make it possible for human beings to live indefinitely on this planet. This book, and the activities of Clonaid are stimulating world wide interest and debate in this massively important field of human endeavour.
Claude Rael's earlier books **The Final Message** (ISBN 0-9530921-1-9, £10.00) and **Sensual Meditation** (ISBN 1-903571-07-3, £10.00), which have already sold over a million copies in 24 languages world wide are also available from The Tagman Press.

God is Never Late...But Never Early Either *by Ian Graham*
P'back ISBN 1-903571-01-4 £10.00. Hardback ISBN 1-903571-02-2 £17.50
Already published to acclaim in Germany and The Netherlands and in production in Italy, Brazil and Denmark, this first book by a remarkable Scottish spiritual healer provides strikingly innovative interpretations of human spirituality which are becoming increasingly important in all our lives. 'These teachings should help bring the wave of spiritual questing currently sweeping the world to a new level of awareness, positivity and power', says a major reviewer of a book that is clearly destined to take a prominent place internationally among the very best of modern spiritual writings.

Please address all orders for Tagman Press books and tapes to Tagman Distribution Direct via the credit card telephone hotlines, fax or e mail addresses given at the top of page 177.